Everything a Man Needs to Know to Prevent Hair Loss

DJ Sully

Cover art by Max Sully (www.maxxsart.com)
Thanks to Patty, Matty and Jenny
MEDICAL DISCLAIMER: The following information is intended for general information purposes only. Individuals should always see their health care provider before administering any suggestions made in this book.

CONTENTS

Part 1: Why is my Hair falling out and what can I do about it?

"It's ridiculous, but it's horrible going bald. Anyone who says it isn't is lying." James Nesbitt

Let's face it; most men would do almost anything to stop going bald. Hair is considered one of the most defining aspects of our appearance and an important way we express self-image. The extent to which our lives are affected by hair loss is reflected in the money spent each year on various products, both prescription and alternative, that claim to cure the problem. The industry today is estimated to be worth around $3.5 billion worldwide.[1]

The word 'alopecia' is the general medical term for baldness. *Androgenetic alopecia* (male pattern baldness or MPB) accounts for more than 95 percent of hair loss in men. However, MPB is nothing new. The Ebers Papyrus, an Egyptian medical text dating back to around 1550 BC, offered a number of unusual remedies. Despite plaguing humans for thousands of years, a cure has yet to be found.

Today it is widely believed that hair loss is either incurable or that nothing can prevent it except pharmaceuticals. Despite what you may have heard, various natural ingredients and lifestyle changes have proven to be significantly more successful than the best-selling hair loss medication. But there are reasons why these choices are not well known.

Firstly, these products and methods cannot be patented, so they will never go through any clinical trials. This means they will not be 'approved' to prevent hair loss or have any legal claims to their effectiveness. Also they will never be promoted nor widely advertised, as companies cannot profit from them. Secondly, they usually require effort, time and commitment to take effect. There is no quick or simple natural solution. For some men it is far easier to use drugs or have surgery than deal with the underlying problems. Lastly, as hair loss is multi-factorial, there cannot be one solution to the problem, natural or otherwise. Several issues need to be addressed. What works for me might not work for you. There is no single answer for all men.

This book provides a science-based, proactive, long-term and holistic approach to attain healthy looking hair and to prevent further loss. A holistic outlook involves thinking about the bigger picture and fixing the causes of the issue, not just relieving the symptoms. What we call symptoms are just surface expressions of what's going on at a much deeper level. These less obvious reasons are what need to be addressed. If there were an easy way to stop hair loss from happening, we would already know about it.

If you do not wish to use any pharmaceutical drugs or resort to any drastic procedures such as surgery but would prefer to take responsibility for your own health, then this is the book for you. I will share with you various ways that have been tested and verified to improve hair growth and tell you how to use this information in your daily life.

- Why drugs or surgery are not your only options
- Why the hormone DHT is not the main reason for your hair loss
- What blood tests you need to identify any specific issues
- Common nutritional deficiencies that can affect your hair growth
- How to increase your levels of testosterone and balance other hormonal systems
- What foods you should be eating and those that should be avoided
- Which herbs have been shown to increase hair growth
- What products to use on your hair and which ones to throw in the bin
- The hidden sources of toxin exposure that are contributing to your problem
- Why certain medical conditions are associated with hair loss
- Why stress whether chemical, emotional or physical is a potential source of hair loss and how to decrease it
- Which natural remedies have outperformed pharmaceutical drugs
- All recent scientific research on hair loss and what it means for you

What Causes Hair Loss?

"No one can overcome a health problem using the same mind-set that created the problem." Thomas Edison

Whether you realise it or not, your hair loss has been earned, though you might not have been directly responsible for all of the causes. Our bodies follow biological laws of causation. What we put into them and how we treat them is directly reflected in our health. This book can be summarized into one simple idea: your hair loss has developed through years of various stresses being put on your system.

If you eat doughnuts for breakfast; drink three cans of soda a day; consume fast and processed food all the time; indulge in excess alcohol; take medicinal and recreational drugs indiscriminately; expose yourself to toxic substances; smoke; rarely exercise and are overweight; put yourself under chronic stress; spend most of the day inside behind a desk; surround yourself with electronics; not get sufficient rest, then it is simply ridiculous to either blame a member of your family, believe you are sensitive to some hormone, or just take another drug. Yet that is what the vast majority of men do. The biggest problem is that our lives are very different from what we were naturally designed to lead. There is some serious disconnect between our evolutionary needs and our modern way of life. What we really need is a shift in perspective.

Are Genes the Cause of Hair Loss? Am I doomed, no matter what I do?

"Genes tell us what may happen, but not if or how." T. Colin Campbell, *Whole*

Some men are physiologically predisposed to hair loss and receding hair lines much more than others. Your genetic code only determines your susceptibility: it does not mean that it's inevitable. Even if you were born with a natural tendency to lose your hair, your family history does not have to become your personal destiny. We all have our inherited weaknesses: it is these flaws that determine which disease or problem will occur as our body is exposed to stresses as we go through life. Some genetic aspects determine an individual's propensity to this issue but they will only occur when

7

these stresses are present. It is not the genes themselves that cause hair loss.

In the words of author Dr Jeffrey S. Bland: *"Throughout your life the most profound influences on your health, vitality and function are not the doctors you have visited or the drugs, surgery or other therapies you have undertaken. The most profound influences are the cumulative effects of the decisions you make about your diet and lifestyle on the expression of your genes."* When you think of your inherited genetic code, you probably think about what kinds of characteristics and risk factors your parents passed on to you through their own DNA. For many years it was thought that this genetic code couldn't be changed. Now we know that even though the genes encoded by DNA are essentially static, the expression of those genes can be highly dynamic.

The relatively new scientific field 'epigenetics' refers to natural control mechanisms that influence gene expression without changing DNA. Non-genetic factors such as diet, chronic stress, lifestyle and environmental factors can change the ways our genes express themselves. These epigenetic changes can be permanent or temporary. In other words, it is not our genes that will cause our hair to fall out even if we are predisposed to the condition but rather external factors over which we have control such as our diet and exposure to toxins that act upon and express these genes. In the words of nutritionist Judith Stern: "*Genetics loads the gun, but environment pulls the trigger.*" Though this basic idea is generally accepted for conditions such as diabetes and heart disease, it is still widely denied with regard to MPB. If you have started losing your hair while other members of your family have already done so, then in some ways it makes sense to blame genetics and feel it is inevitable. By a similar argument, you are probably sharing a high degree of behavioural and environmental similarity with other family members. Genetics is not the only scapegoat.

The ancient Greek physician Hippocrates recognised a connection between sexual organs and baldness, noting that if eunuchs were castrated before puberty they did not go bald however strong the familial disposition. However, if they were castrated during or after puberty, they lost their hair just as other men did. More recent studies have shown that genetically identical twins can lose their hair at very different rates, despite being born with the same genes.[2,3] Clearly, there is something more to the picture than just genetics.

Is DHT to Blame?
"The worst thing a man can do is go bald." Donald Trump

The other mainstream theory is that the male hormone DHT (dihydrotestosterone) is the singular evil with regard to MPB. From research conducted in the 1940s by Dr James Hamilton, it was discovered that castrated men were presumably protected from baldness because of their lack of testosterone. It was also noted they had noticeably less oily hair and skin, as well as less dandruff. He injected them with testosterone propionate and noticed that in a limited number their hair subsequently fell out. Then in 1974, Dr Julianne Imperato-McGinley studied twenty-four male pseudo-hermaphrodites (men with incomplete masculinization of the external genitalia) who had normal levels of testosterone though also had no signs of hair loss. The pseudo-hermaphrodites were determined to be deficient in an enzyme (5-alpha reductase) that converts testosterone to DHT. The researchers then concluded it was not testosterone but DHT that was responsible for MPB.

The current medical consensus is that DHT, along with a genetic predisposition, causes hair loss and this is known as the 'androgen theory.' The general idea is that DHT accumulates in the scalp, binds to hair follicles activating the androgen receptors, causing them to shrink and stop producing hair. There are several observations to back up this theory: men born with a genetic deficiency in DHT never go bald; finasteride is a drug that lowers DHT levels and can delay the progression of MPB in some men; women typically have a far lower level of this hormone and consequently suffer less from hair loss; and DHT has been found to accumulate in the scalps of men with MPB.

These findings make it clear that there is indeed a link between DHT and hair loss but there are a number of fundamental flaws to this theory: most notably the lack of an explanation of why levels increase in the scalp in the first place; it does not answer how this hormone causes hair growth elsewhere on the body but is supposed to do the complete opposite in certain areas on the scalp; men who are not losing their hair typically have higher circulating levels of DHT; if this hormone alone were the cause of MPB then any drug that reduced levels should be effective in all men; no explanation for the rising incidence of hair loss in younger men; as we age our levels of androgens decrease but older men suffer more from hair loss; no valid explanation to more current observations that involve various inflammatory chemicals; and finally it does not address known causes of hair loss such as nutritional deficiencies or drug-induced hair loss.[4] Obviously something more is happening than merely increased levels or sensitivity to DHT.

Dr James Hamilton noted contradictions in his own findings, saying: *"The suspicion arises that androgens are not the 'directly causative' agent in baldness, but only one member- albeit a frequently effective one- of a family of remote causes that affect local areas capable of reacting in a special manner."* The androgen theory is based on studies of castrates and later on pseudo-hermaphrodites, both of whom have vastly different hormonal profiles compared to typical men. Castrates, for example, are also deficient in the hormones oestrogen and prolactin while pseudo-hermaphrodites have low DHT levels in both their blood and scalp tissues.

It is well documented that androgens including DHT are critically important for sexual function and development of genitalia in men. Patients with erectile dysfunction treated with DHT can show improvement in function and libido and yet some hair loss drugs are doing just the opposite. Not surprising then that a common side effect from the popular medication finasteride (marketed as Propecia and Proscar) is a reduction in libido and erectile dysfunction. These effects can last for several years even after the medication has been discontinued. I do not think it is a good idea to attempt to mimic the androgen profile of a pseudo-hermaphrodite although this is the object behind such drugs. Reducing the production of DHT does not stop the primary cause of your hair loss. We need to prevent whatever is causing this androgen to accumulate in the scalp in the first place.

Both your genes and DHT are involved with your hair loss but neither is likely to be the main causative factor. A lot of research assumes the androgen theory is correct and fits their results into that framework, even if the evidence is obviously conflicting. Unfortunately, the idea that DHT is solely responsible for MPB is the reason behind best-selling hair loss medications.

For more information about the history of research into this subject, I thoroughly recommend Danny Roddy's book *Hair Like a Fox,* plus videos on his website www.dannyroddy.com. He also highlights that DHT is not solely responsible for MPB and that the androgen theory is completely invalid.

Rugs, Plugs or Drugs? Getting to the Root of the Problem Instead

"It isn't simply vanity – most people do look worse without hair."
Alain de Botton

Today the most common solution is pharmaceutical drugs, despite the realities of some hideous side effects, lifelong commitment and, for many, lack of success. Apart from medication another popular treatment is a follicular hair transplant (hair plugs). These can cost more than $50,000 and may have to be repeated a few years later. This invasive surgery also carries the possibility of complications such as death of cells at the donor site, irregular scar tissue formation and inflammation of hair follicles. Other popular solutions include laser therapy, platelet-rich plasma injections, botox injections, wearing a hairpiece or just shaving off what hair remains. Most importantly, all fail to address the causes of the problem.

It's a natural tendency for people to try to find easy fixes to their problems. Simplistic answers and solutions are satisfying but, unfortunately, they are usually inadequate. There is no meaningful way to reduce hair loss to a solitary source. It is exactly this sort of reductionist thinking that sells drugs and makes headlines. We tend to think linearly and look for singular cause and effects but hair loss is a staggeringly complex set of processes and interactions. You can't merely name one contributing factor and ignore all the rest. The idea of having too much of one hormone in the scalp as being the only cause of this problem is an inaccurate oversimplification. There are multiple reasons why men suffer hair loss just as there are numerous explanations why we have other health problems. The question you should be asking is not what leads to hair loss but rather what combination of factors is causing *my* hair loss.

Rather than taking an honest and hard look at what is possibly giving rise to their hair loss, many men are still seeking a miraculous cure. They want to believe that, in spite of all their indiscretions and excesses, they can still maintain optimal health by using a pill, powder or lotion. If you are looking for a simple fix to such a complex problem then you will eventually be disappointed. Hair loss is a multi-factorial condition that apart from a genetic predisposition can be owing to: hormones and nutrient imbalances; toxin exposure and accumulation; inflammation and oxidative stress; health of your body systems and general state of health; levels of physical activity; medications you may be taking and how you treat your hair. These aspects are interrelated. There is some disconnect that treats MPB as a divergent condition seemingly totally separate from these known causes of hair loss.

Is Your Hair Giving You Early Warning Signals About Your Health?

"Baldness is not a disease or even a medical problem per se, yet it seems to be an early warning sign that other problems may loom in the future." Dr Charles J. Ryan, *The Virility Paradox*

Although most doctors don't regard hair loss as a major concern, it may have more than just psychological or cosmetic implications. Researchers have found that men who have MPB have higher rates of heart disease, hypertension (high blood pressure), diabetes and pre-diabetes, prostate cancer, obesity and poor libido. Here are a few examples of some recent scientific studies:

•A 2017 study revealed that men under forty years that had MPB and prematurely greying hair had more than five times the normal rate of suffering from heart disease.[5] This represents a risk higher than one posed by obesity. Hair loss without greying raised the risk by three times. The research found that the greater the severity of hair loss equated to an increase in the threat of heart disease. Dr Sharma, the principal researcher on the study, stated: "*Baldness and premature graying should be considered risk factors for coronary artery disease. These factors may indicate biological, rather than chronological, age which may be important in determining total cardiovascular risk.*" 800 men with heart disease and 1,270 healthy relatives were investigated.

•In a 2007 study researchers found MPB was "*strongly associated with hypertension.*"[6] Men with blood pressure higher than 120 over 80 had twice the risk of hair loss compared to those with lower readings. 250 men aged thirty-five to sixty-five were examined.

•A 2013 meta-analysis (a statistical analysis that combines the results of multiple scientific studies) of 8,994 patients found that loss of hair from the crown of the head was associated with a significantly increased risk of prostate cancer.[7]

•A 2010 population-based study from Taiwan recognised a significant association between MPB and metabolic syndrome (pre-diabetes).[8] 740 men aged between forty and ninety-one were surveyed.

•A 2014 study found that a higher body mass index (BMI) was significantly associated with greater severity of hair loss, especially in those with early onset MPB (developing before thirty-five years of age).[9] 189 men with a mean age of just under thirty-one were investigated.

•A 2016 assessment of semen quality in 203 young men with hair loss in an infertility clinic showed that those with moderate to severe MPB had poorer quality of semen compared to men with normal to mild MPB.[10]

Admittedly these studies all show associated rather than causal relationships. They do, however, suggest that hair loss is probably more than follicles being sensitive to DHT.

Prevention is Better than a Non-existent Cure

"Illnesses do not come upon us out of the blue. They are developed from small daily sins against Nature. When enough sins have accumulated, illnesses will suddenly appear." Hippocrates

We need to focus on what we can do to nurture our body on a daily basis rather than waiting for something to go wrong, then expect some drug or procedure to fix it. No one single product either natural or man-made will cure hair loss, although it is much easier to believe in some wonder pill or therapy that will instantly solve the problem with little effort involved. There is no simple remedy for your hair loss. There are just ways to prevent it. Unfortunately, preventions are not as exciting as cures. These take time, self-discipline, a desire to change as well as being able to sacrifice some of your comforts and adjust certain habits.

From his book *Whole* author and biochemist T. Colin Campbell says this: *"Changing one's lifestyle can be challenging. It requires commitment and responsibility from the person making the change, and a willingness to be open to having new experiences and developing new habits and skills. A quick-fix solution is a much easier sale than the long-haul, comprehensive, wholistic solution. There is no incentive for industry to invest in the nutritional effects of certain foods or lifestyle changes, and no incentive for researchers to study and validate such claims."*

To combat such a complicated condition as hair loss, you must begin a strategy that incorporates several different changes into your life: a more multi-layered approach will increase your chances of success. A large body of scientific evidence suggests all of the following can improve hair growth: an excellent and varied diet; regular exercise; stress management; adequate sleep patterns; reducing the intake of toxic chemicals; removal of accumulated toxins from your body and transforming your personal environment. All of these everyday choices when combined have a real impact on the health of your hair. I recognise and appreciate real-world concerns such as lack of time, pressure at work and home, ingrained eating habits and money issues, all of which can disrupt any resolutions you have made.

Some shifts will happen immediately while others take time and may be problematic. For many men, changing what they eat can be extremely challenging, while for others reducing stress at work and at home can be the most difficult. You must make informed and healthier choices every day. You could start out with great enthusiasm and expectations but these resolves may begin to fade over time. New positive habits take time to become ingrained and there are ample opportunities to get off track. Certain habits die hard but they do die.

Hair Growth

"In all forms of alopecia, the hair follicles remain alive and are ready to resume normal hair production whenever they receive the appropriate signal." The National Alopecia Areata Foundation

Next to bone marrow and the lining of your stomach, hair is the fastest growing tissue in the human body. Because of its rapid growth, it is acutely sensitive to internal or external changes. Everyone loses hair from their head every day, usually around forty to one hundred strands, with most of the loss occurring in the morning.

Hair refers to two distinct structures: the part beneath the skin called the hair follicle (hair root), and the hair shaft which extends above the surface. Although people say your hair is dead, that depends on which bit you're referring to. The hair follicle is alive but since the visible shaft doesn't contain any nerves, it is considered nonliving tissue.

By week twenty-two, a developing foetus has all of its hair follicles formed. At this stage somewhere around 100,000 to 150,000 of those reside on the scalp. This is the largest number you will ever have, since we do not generate new ones at any time during the course of our lives. As with other mammals, humans appear to be subject to seasonal differences with growth rates being greater in the summer months. Despite men suffering more from hair loss, ours is thicker and grows faster than female hair.

Hair on the scalp grows in follicular units that produce between two and five follicles that emerge from a single pore. The size of each follicle determines the thickness of the hair shaft and the thinner the hair's diameter then the shorter it grows. Any factor that decreases the size of the follicle will subsequently decrease the width and length of the hair it produces. Men with MPB have smaller follicles. A reduction in the number of hairs per follicular unit also occurs when you begin losing hair. However, if a follicle remains intact, it is possible to regrow or improve the health of the remaining hair. Therefore, yes it is possible to grow back hair on your scalp that has been lost.

At the base of the follicle is the hair bulb that contains numerous structures including the dermal papilla. This is where blood vessels deliver nutrients to the follicle and actively-growing cells continually divide and push upwards, gradually hardening and eventually producing hair. The number of cells in the dermal papilla dictates the size of the hair and may play a crucial role in initiating the formation of a new shaft. When the numbers of these cells fall below a critical threshold, new hairs are not generated.[11] This is also where the receptors for androgens are located, which are known to regulate hair growth.

Another important part of the hair follicle is the sebaceous glands that secrete an oily substance known as sebum. This protects your hair from the elements and acts as a barrier against foreign agents such as bacteria and viruses. Sebum seals in the hair's moisture and lubricates it externally, keeping friction and wear at a minimum. It also gives hair elasticity and flexibility. Men with MPB have been shown to have enlarged sebaceous glands and increased sebum production.[12]

Each hair follows a specific growth cycle with three distinct phases: anagen, catagen and telogen. While the stages always progress in the same order, different hairs on your head are going through separate phases concurrently. The signals that induce the transition between these different phases of the hair cycle are not completely understood though many modulators, hormones and growth factors have been identified.

At any given time, about 90 percent of your hair is actively growing. This growth phase, known as anagen, when the cells in the follicle are dividing rapidly, can last for two to seven years, though the average is about three. During this stage, hair typically grows around one centimetre every month. The proportion of follicles in this growth period declines with age and in men experiencing hair loss. Hair follicles may exit the anagen phase owing to illness, trauma, physical and emotional stress, or because of some metabolic change.

At the end of the growth period is a short regression stage, known as the catagen phase, which lasts only a few weeks. This is when the hair follicle detaches from the dermal papilla, blood supply is cut and the follicle begins shrinking.

The final stage, known as telogen, is when growth stops and the shaft is released (this shedding is also known as exogen). In a healthy scalp this resting or dormant stage lasts around three to five months and is happening to about 10 percent of hair. Energy metabolism in the follicles increases during the transition from telogen to the anagen phase as a new shaft begins to grow and the cycle starts again. If there is a disturbance in the delivery of glucose at this transition time then anagen may be delayed. Glucose is one of the main fuels for the hair follicle, especially at this stage.[13]

In MPB, the growth phase decreases with each hair cycle, while the length of the resting phase remains constant or is prolonged. Ultimately, the growth phase becomes so short that the growing hair fails to achieve sufficient length to reach the surface of the skin.

What we think of as hair loss can be better described as a miniaturization (shrinking) of the follicle. Several scientific studies will be discussed throughout the book that show certain substances either increasing the growth phase and leading to less hair being lost or shortening the growth phase and ultimately causing more hair to be lost.

Part 2: Hormones, Inflammation and Modulators

"Aside from androgens, hair follicles express receptors for estrogens, cortisol, retinoids, insulin, thyroid hormones, vitamin D, and many other known and unknown factors – the full influence of which is still being investigated, but points to the fact that these affect intrinsic signaling pathways and that a balance of all is what ultimately determines hair growth." New Insight into the Pathophysiology of Hair Loss Trigger a Paradigm Shift in the Treatment Approach

Before I advise you to remove your fillings; cease taking a daily multivitamin; throw your shampoo and deodorant in the bin; stop drinking out of plastic bottles; start eating seaweed and sauerkraut; sleep in a dark room and spend more time in the sun, it's good to know why I recommend seemingly random and totally unconnected actions with regard to hair loss. To do that we first need to look in detail at possible reasons for your problem, which may include hormonal and nutritional imbalances, inflammation and oxidative stress: and why you need to adapt your diet and lifestyle to affect them positively.

HORMONES

"...no hormone works in isolation. All of these fascinating substances interact with and influence each other, which is why a spike in one hormone typically causes a drop in another. This complex interplay is part of the body's incredible mechanism for coping with an imbalanced state. Too much or too little of any one hormone can interfere with your metabolism, accelerate aging, and compromise your overall wellness." Natasha Turner, *The Hormone Diet*

Hormones are powerful chemical messengers created by the body. They are used in minute amounts in extremely intricate ways to control most major bodily functions, from simple basic needs such as hunger and sleep to complex systems like reproduction and even your emotions and mood. Each sex has highly significant quantities of the opposite sex's major sex hormone in their bodies.

Both male and female hormones affect hair growth and play an important role in its health and quality. However, it is the elaborate interaction of several hormones and not just sex hormones that affect our hair.

Imbalances lead to several health issues including hair loss. The good news is that any dysfunction can be addressed through diet and lifestyle changes. However, this is not something that can be achieved overnight. A healthy diet is essential for keeping your hormones balanced and poor nutritional habits are a major cause of imbalance. Other factors that need to be addressed include your levels of stress, exercise and sleep patterns, liver function, digestive health and exposure to toxins.

Understanding how certain hormones affect our body is important. We can adjust our eating habits and lifestyles to increase the amounts of some while decreasing the levels of others. Some of the major hormones involved in hair growth are: testosterone, DHT, oestrogen, thyroid hormone, prolactin, cortisol and insulin. Owing to their effects on hair, they can be thought of as either 'positive' or 'negative'. As there is considerable crossover in their imbalances, you will probably have to adjust the levels of several hormones rather than just focusing on any individual one.

Keeping Your Mojo: Testosterone, DHT and SHBG

"...men should be concerned about declining total testosterone, even if it has not reached a level to warrant a clinical diagnosis...A lot of men may not be aware of the risk factors for testosterone deficiency because of their current lifestyle." Dr Mark Peterson

Male sexual hormones are collectively known as androgens and include testosterone and DHT. Androgens stimulate hair growth on the face and body and create fuller, thicker hair on the head. Testosterone is mainly produced by Leydig cells in the testicles but is also produced in small amounts by the adrenal glands. The enzyme 5-alpha reductase irreversibly converts this hormone to DHT. Almost 10 percent of the testosterone produced by men each day is changed to DHT by the testes and prostate. This androgen is particularly potent, about five or so times more powerful than testosterone.

Testosterone travels to every part of your body and is responsible for the biological characteristics that typify males: our deep voice, body shape, muscle mass, sperm production, odour in the form of pheromones, hairiness as well as typical male behaviour like dominance, assertiveness and sex drive. It also controls both our vitality and longevity. Its production increases when we are aroused and feel we are succeeding in life. Alternatively when stressed, bored or feel we are losing in life, our levels decrease. Men who maintain higher amounts as they age have significantly less heart disease and fewer symptoms of mental senility compared to those with low levels. One study found that men with the lowest amounts of testosterone had a 40 percent elevated risk of dying from any cause compared to those with the highest amounts.[1]

Increasing and maintaining testosterone levels is extremely beneficial for your general health as well as for your hair. Unfortunately, it's not so simple just to increase this hormone and your hair won't fall out. It is only one of the factors that come into play. Many of the effects that this hormone has in the body only happen after it is converted to DHT. This potent androgen supports sexual function and libido; aids feelings of well-being; increases lean muscle and strength; enhances the ability of the body to lower blood sugar levels; reduces body fat; and is responsible for the growth and thickness of hair. If you block DHT production, then any of these factors could be negatively impacted.

In a 2014 study researchers measured DHT levels in patients with hair loss (nineteen women and nine men) and concluded that: *"The differences in mean values of DHT were not significant according to the types of alopecia and the control group. Increased serum (blood) concentrations of DHT were not correlated with the advance of alopecia* [MPB]."[2]

Although increased circulating levels of DHT are, therefore, not the cause of your hair loss, tissue levels of this hormone in balding areas have been found to be higher than non-balding areas.[3] The androgenic theory assumes every hair follicle on your scalp is genetically predisposed to be susceptible to DHT. Unfortunately, this does not answer the critical question of why it accumulates there in the first place. Obviously, it is not the start of hair loss, so we need to find out under what circumstances this androgen could collect in the scalp tissues.

Various studies have shown inflammation and several pro-inflammatory markers are inhibited by DHT.[4,5,6] Therefore, higher levels are detectable in the scalps of men with MPB not because it is the cause of hair loss but rather a symptom of chronic inflammation. Oxidative stress has also been shown to increase levels of DHT in the dermal papilla cells of the scalp.[7] Inflammation and oxidative stress are probable causes of your hair loss not DHT. As we will see soon, the presence of both has been found in the scalps of men with hair loss.

You should avoid all 5-alpha reductase inhibitors (the enzyme that converts testosterone to DHT) as you do *not* want to inhibit the production of DHT. These include hair loss drugs that contain finasteride which decreases both blood and tissue levels of this hormone. Even though you might have decreasing scalp levels of DHT and increasing testosterone in your body, it would be at the expense of reducing total DHT, which results in an overall negative effect on your androgen level. To get the maximum benefits out of your testosterone, make sure it naturally converts into DHT and is not blocked. You want to decrease levels of this androgen in the scalp but not at the expense of reducing it in the rest of your body.

An important factor to consider when discussing your androgen levels is SHBG. Sex hormone binding globulin is primarily produced in the liver and attaches to sex hormones including testosterone, DHT and oestrogen. It transports them throughout the body and regulates a healthy balance between a man's testosterone and oestrogen levels. Most testosterone circulating in your bloodstream is bound either to SHBG or another protein, albumin. Total testosterone measures that which is bound to these two proteins and that which is not. Any hormone attached to SHBG is essentially 'locked up' and not available for use. The availability of testosterone is therefore influenced by your level of SHBG. Only a small fraction (around 1 to 3 percent) is unbound or 'free' to enter a cell and activate its receptor. Free testosterone is completely biologically available and is the most relevant measure of a man's testosterone status. It is your hormonal gold.

Your SHBG should be within the healthy range, and the only way to find out is to get tested. Neither a high nor low level is what you want. Factors that increase SHBG will reduce free testosterone and therefore can be considered bad for the health of your hair. At the same time, a low level is also an unhealthy sign and indicates other issues.

A 2004 study looked at the hormonal profile of thirty-seven men with MPB. The frequency of subnormal values in SHBG was significant in those balding.[8] Younger men who are suffering from MPB generally have lower levels of SHBG compared with those the same age without hair loss. This should mean higher free testosterone but other factors come into play. Lower levels in men with MPB are a sign of reduced thyroid hormones, chronic inflammation, obesity and insulin resistance.

A later 2011 study examined 120 patients with early onset MPB (sixty men and sixty women) and the researchers concluded that: *"An association between early-onset AGA [MPB], hyperglycemia/diabetes, and low levels of SHBG was observed in the current study. Low levels of SHBG could be a marker of insulin resistance and hyperglycemia/diabetes in patients with AGA."*[9] Low circulating levels of SHBG are a strong predictor of the risk of type 2 diabetes as well as for early onset hair loss.

If your SHBG levels are too high, then you need to focus on raising your testosterone while lowering oestrogen and cortisol. Alternately, if they are too low, lose weight if you are overweight; exercise more often;[10] enhance thyroid function; improve insulin sensitivity; reduce inflammation; and boost the health of your liver.

How to Avoid Low Androgen Levels

The unsexy truth is that naturally increasing testosterone and DHT comes down to making long-term changes in your diet and lifestyle and these are discussed throughout the book. They include exercising and changing your body mass, improving your diet, reducing stress and toxin exposure, as well as adjusting your sleep patterns. Use of drugs, both recreational and pharmaceutical, including marijuana, steroids, opiates, alcohol, ibuprofen, acetaminophen (paracetamol) and antacids may possibly lower androgen levels. Increasing androgens also means adjusting the levels of other hormones. These processes are intertwined and all need to be addressed rather than focusing on a single issue.

Testosterone levels do not necessarily decline with age. It is commonly reported that after the age of forty, levels typically fall around 1.5 percent per year. A review found: *"no evidence for a further fall in mean total testosterone with increasing age through to old age. However we do show that there is an increased variation in total testosterone levels with advancing age after age 40 years.*"[11] This decline rather than being a direct result of age itself is more likely to be from nutrition, lifestyle and exercise choices. These become more apparent and significant as time passes. Substantial variability in testosterone levels in different men is responsible rather than an inevitable small decrease each year as we become older.

A 2013 study, known as 'The Finnish Study,' reported that a man born in 1970 has 20 percent less testosterone than his father did at the same age.[12] The researchers offered no explanation but exposure to chemical oestrogens, nutrient deficiencies, certain medications and lack of physical activity are all probable causes. The increases in our exposure to oestrogen and oestrogen-like substances are highly significant in explaining these generational decreases in testosterone.

Getting Tested for Testosterone and SHBG

The only way to really know what your hormone levels are is to get tested. One problem is there hasn't been much standardization in hormone testing, particularly regarding testosterone. Different labs use different methods and measurements. When you get checked, there are two main tests to get: total testosterone and free testosterone. While the US generally uses nanograms/decilitre (ng/dL) and picograms/millilitre (pg/mL) other countries use nanomoles/litre (nmol/L) and picomoles/litre (pmol/L). You can apply one of the many conversion tables found online to convert results. A normal level will depend on how old you are though many labs don't break down reference ranges by age. Here is a general guide:

Test	Reference
Total Testosterone	18-39 years: 350-1080 ng/dL 40-59 years: 350-890 ng/dL 60 years and older: 300-720 ng/dL
Free Testosterone	18 years and older: 47-244 pg/mL
Percentage Free Testosterone	18 years and older: 1.6-2.9 %

Another problem is that different laboratories don't agree on reference ranges. These are very wide as they encompass the 'normal' range for adult men of all ages. A target number of 700 ng/dL or higher for total testosterone is what you should ideally be aiming for if you are under forty. For all three readings in the table it is preferable to have results at the higher end of the reference range.

While blood tests are much more accurate and sensitive than saliva or urine tests, they're also more expensive. It's best to get your blood drawn first thing in the morning as testosterone levels are at their highest in the morning and steadily decline throughout the day. To measure your total testosterone, try finding the LC/MS test. It's more accurate than ECLIA. To measure your free testosterone, the Equilibrium Ultrafiltration test is more reliable than RIA Direct. Calculated free testosterone is the least accurate way. Some doctors suggest that monitoring testosterone levels every five years, starting at age thirty-five, is a reasonable strategy to follow.

SHBG: The normal ranges for men are 10-57 nmol/L. Ideally, you want to have a reading somewhere around 28-32 nmol/L.

For a full male hormone panel, you can also test: oestradiol, androstenedione, DHEA, DHT, lutenizing hormone and cortisol levels. As with all tests, ask your doctor to go over the results with you.

Oestrogen

Oestrogen (also known as estrogen) isn't a single hormone but a group of steroid hormones and their bioactive metabolites with oestradiol being the most potent form. Whilst women have the most, men do possess some as it is critical for healthy bones, sexual functioning, skin health, blood flow and brain function. Oestrogen and testosterone need to stay in balance for good health. If you have low testosterone then you will have elevated amounts of oestrogen. It is not possible to have either high or low level of both hormones at the same time. As we want our testosterone as high as we can naturally get, then it is necessary to decrease oestrogen as much as possible. This is an extremely important part in maintaining our hormonal balance and preventing hair loss.

In a 2006 study researchers stated: *"Androgens are recognized key regulators of normal human hair growth and the prerequisite for sexual hair and sebaceous gland development. However, estrogens also profoundly alter hair growth in practically all mammalian species investigated."*[13] As opposed to androgens, oestrogen acts primarily as an inhibitor to hair growth and so it's definitely one of the enemies of your hair.

In an earlier 1996 study topical treatment of oestrogen on mice arrested follicles in the resting phase and produced a profound and prolonged inhibition of hair growth.[14] Alternately, topical treatments with an oestrogen receptor antagonist caused follicles to exit the resting phase and enter the growth stage. Oestrogen caused hair loss while a substance opposing the actions of this hormone increased growth.

Levels of this hormone can be elevated in men with MPB. A 1991 study examined sixty-five men with hair loss.[15] Significant differences in the levels of oestrogen compared to control subjects were found.

Women synthesize most of this hormone in their ovaries and since men lack this female anatomy, we need to produce it another way. We achieve it through a natural process involving an enzyme called aromatase that transforms testosterone (but not DHT) into oestrogen. In one study sixteen men were given an aromatase inhibitor for eight weeks.[16] Levels of free testosterone, DHT and the ratio of testosterone to oestrogen were all significantly increased. Therefore, blocking the formation of oestrogen will produce an increase in androgen levels.

As we want to decrease our levels of oestrogen, it is important to prevent the actions of aromatase as much as possible. Rather than taking any drugs, there are many ways to naturally reduce this enzyme without any side effects. Aromatase can be inhibited by consuming foods rich in zinc, magnesium and selenium (all three are common deficiencies). Celery, nettle root and cruciferous vegetables such as broccoli as well as foods containing the phytonutrients luteolin, quercetin, apigenin and naringenin (refer to part 3 for more information on phytonutrients) also help in reducing activity.

An excess of oestrogen has several other negative effects within the body that can contribute to hair loss aside from reducing androgen levels. It also tampers with thyroid hormone, increases both prolactin and cortisol levels, modulates the release of inflammatory chemicals and interferes with glucose metabolism contributing to insulin resistance.[17]

Apart from the natural conversion, there are external sources of oestrogen that need to be considered. Whether aware of it or not, you are constantly exposed to chemicals both natural and synthetic that have a similar effect on the body as this hormone. They are found in the air, water and food, pharmaceutical drugs and products you put on your body and use around the house. These chemicals act together to produce cumulative and powerful effects. Never have we been exposed to such an overwhelming amount of these oestrogen-like substances.

Xenoestrogens

Endocrine disruptors are chemicals that interfere with the body's endocrine system and produce adverse effects. A wide range of substances, both natural and man-made, are thought to alter the normal function of hormones. Xenoestrogens (foreign oestrogens) are a sub-category of these endocrine disruptors that specifically have oestrogen-like effects. The oestrogen receptor in the body is nonspecific enough to permit binding with a diverse array of these chemical structures. Xenoestrogens can also bind directly to androgen receptors, thus blocking androgens from binding and having an effect. When xenoestrogens enter the body, they increase the overall activity of oestrogen and subsequently decrease the overall activity of testosterone and other androgens.

There are three kinds of xenoestrogens: those found in plants (phytoestrogens); those created synthetically in the laboratory (synthetic xenoestrogens); and those found in fungi (mycoestrogens).

Phytoestrogens

These are found in many different plants and, potentially, can have an oestrogen-like effect on your body. Just because a food or herb contains these compounds, you shouldn't automatically avoid it. Many foods that contain phytoestrogens are excellent for your hair. The goal is to eliminate only the most potent ones from your diet. 121 foods were investigated and by far and away the highest concentration by several magnitudes was found in flax and soy, as well as their by-products.[18] In regards to phytoestrogens, just try avoiding these two products. This is more easily said than done as both are present in many foods especially processed foods and cooking oils.

Synthetic Xenoestrogens

Many man-made chemicals ubiquitous in the environment disrupt our endocrine system one way or another. Synthetic xenoestrogens imitate the effects of oestrogen and are much more potent than what your body makes or those found in food. The body is able to break down and excrete phytoestrogens relatively easily, while many of the synthetic xenoestrogens resist breakdown and accumulate, exposing us to low-level but long-term exposure. They can persist for many years, stored in our fat cells.

We want to limit our exposure to these synthetic foreign oestrogens as much as possible. In addition to this, we must actively find ways to remove these toxins stored in our bodies. Common synthetic xenoestrogens are found in plastics, personal-care products, cleaning items as well as pharmaceutical drugs. Various ways to decrease your exposure and how to safely eliminate them from the body will be discussed in part 6.

Mycoestrogens

Like many plants, fungi can also produce oestrogenic compounds, known as mycoestrogens. Zearalenone (ZEA) is a mycoestrogen and also happens to be the most common mould toxin (mycotoxin). Estimates are somewhere around 25 percent of the food crops in the world are affected by various mycotoxins. A number of countries have established legal limits for ZEA levels in food but not the US. There are numerous negative health effects caused by ZEA and other mycotoxins, including increasing oestrogen levels in the body.

In one review researchers concluded that: *"There is no doubt that ZEA and some of its reductive metabolites...are highly active nonsteroidal estrogens with hormonal activities exceeding than that of most phytoestrogens and close to the potency of the mammalian steroidal estrogen E2."*[19] Simply put, ZEA can have effects almost as strong as oestradiol itself. Another review found that feeding young male pigs with contaminated feed containing ZEA resulted in: animals with a testicular weight significantly lower than controls, reduced libido and a decrease in testosterone.[20]

Crops frequently contaminated, either before or after harvest, include cereals (corn, wheat and rice), oilseeds (soybean, peanut, sunflower and cotton seeds), spices (chili peppers, black pepper, coriander, turmeric and ginger), coffee beans, cocoa and tree nuts (pistachio, almond, walnut, coconut and Brazil nut). It is important to note that mould that produces mycotoxins can penetrate deep into food and does not merely grow on the surface. These toxins can travel up the food chain to grain and corn-fed meat, eggs and dairy products.

To minimize the health risk from mycotoxins in these foods, buy grains, spices and nuts as fresh as possible; do not keep these foods for extended periods of time and make sure they are stored properly; soak all grains and nuts before use; do not use seed oils; avoid all grain or corn-fed animal produce; do not eat refined wheat and corn products; keep away from cheap coffee and cheap chocolate. Conversely, eating certain foods can help remove any mycotoxins in your digestive system: foods high in vitamin C, radishes, fresh turmeric root as well as activated charcoal and bentonite clay.

How to Avoid Elevated Oestrogen
Many other factors that increase both aromatase and oestrogen levels will be discussed throughout the book. Liver detoxification is critically important to the breakdown and elimination of this hormone and the body requires sufficient nutrients including zinc, magnesium and selenium to support this process. A steady supply of glucose is also required for its excretion and bacteria in the digestive tract play an important role.

Part of an overall plan to decrease oestrogen in the body should involve: increasing your androgen levels and thyroid function; improving liver and gut health; reducing your contact with synthetic oestrogens and other toxins; lowering your intake of all unfermented soy and flax products; minimizing your exposure to ZEA and lowering your stress levels. In addition, you can remove xenoestrogens stored in your body through fasting.

Getting Tested for Oestrogen
Oestradiol should be between 22-30 pg/mL. The most accurate test is LC/MS-MS. Elevated levels of oestrogen are typically found in men with increased abdominal obesity. By testing your testosterone, you are indirectly measuring your levels of oestrogens,

so this test is not necessary. There is no convenient blood test for measuring xenoestrogens.

Thyroid Hormone

The thyroid gland is found at the front of your neck below the Adam's apple. If it isn't working well, nothing in your body functions effectively. The thyroid produces two hormones that control your metabolism and help to ensure oxygen and glucose get into cells. Anything that decreases thyroid hormone production will reduce the quantity of oxygen and glucose being delivered to the hair follicles. The more active thyroid hormone (synthesized predominantly in the liver) is essential for the development and maintenance of hair follicles. Thyroid hormone is definitely one of your friends with regard to hair growth.

In a 2008 study thyroid hormone was shown to increase the growth phase of the human hair follicle.[21] Conversely, low thyroid function is associated with an increase in the percentage of hair follicles in the resting phase.

Thyroid hormone deficiency negatively alters levels of both cortisol and free testosterone.[22] This hormone also activates various antioxidants that help to reduce oxidative stress.[23] A low functioning thyroid will not only reduce antioxidant activity in the body but also lead to an increase in inflammatory modulators such as TGF-beta1 (known to cause hair loss). This in turn leads to even higher levels of oxidative stress.

The most common cause of insufficient thyroid hormone production is iodine deficiency. This mineral is crucial and, without iodine, you cannot make active thyroid hormone. Selenium, zinc, iron and vitamin A also help to ensure a healthy thyroid gland. All are common deficiencies.

How to Avoid Low Thyroid Hormone
Sea vegetables should be at the top of your list of foods for your thyroid as they are an excellent source of iodine and other minerals. There is a lot written about the negative impact that cruciferous vegetables such as Brussels sprouts, cauliflower and broccoli have on thyroid health. They contain goitrogens which can block iodine from entering the thyroid leading to a deficiency. However, you

would need to eat a large number of these vegetables and they would have to be raw. Also, goitrogens are more likely to negatively impact people who already have poor thyroid function. Cruciferous vegetables are nutritionally dense foods and are good for your thyroid and general health. Wild fish, raw fermented vegetables, green leafy vegetables, radish, Brazil nuts and the herb ashwagandha are also all beneficial for healthy thyroid hormone production. On the other hand, there are certain foods that should be avoided: unfermented soy, polyunsaturated oils, conventional dairy products and gluten. All of these have been shown to interfere negatively with thyroid hormones.

Many other factors negatively affect the creation, transport and activation of thyroid hormones. These include an altered gut microbiome, high oestrogen levels, stress, inflammation, a poorly-functioning liver, as well as environmental toxins such as mercury, fluoride and xenoestrogens.

Getting Your Thyroid Tested

A few tests are required to assess accurately the function of your thyroid gland:

Thyroid-stimulating hormone (TSH): Optimal range should be between 0.5 to 2.0 mU/L. Many younger men with hair loss have a higher level of TSH suggesting increased cortisol and/or prolactin.

Total T4; Free T4; Total T3; Free T3; Reverse T3(rT3); and thyroid antibodies: Readings should be in the middle of your lab's reference range. Elevated reverse T3 usually indicates high levels of stress. Thyroid antibodies should be negative. Free T3 is not part of a regular thyroid panel.

Prolactin

The hormone prolactin is produced by the pituitary gland and is best known for its role in breast milk production (pro-lactation) though men do possess some. In mammals, it has been called the 'moulting hormone' for its well-known ability to shed old feathers, hair or skin. A 2016 study examined the hormone profile of fifty-seven men with early onset MPB.[24] Prolactin levels were significantly increased in men with MPB compared to controls. This hormone is another enemy of your hair.

In one 2009 review researchers found that prolactin retards the entry of follicles into the growth phase, inhibits hair shaft elongation and stimulates excess sebum production.[25] They also discovered that this hormone is one of the major hormonal signals that increase in response to emotional and physical stress; secretion is stimulated by prostaglandins as part of the inflammatory response and inhibits 5-alpha reductase (the enzyme that converts testosterone to DHT) activity *in vitro*. They concluded that: "*...current evidence suggests that* [prolactin] *primarily serves as a hair growth-inhibitory hormone, both in mice and man.*" This hormone is an inhibitor of hair growth and yet *decreases* the production of DHT. The researchers go on to say that: "*Patients with...hair loss disorders may indeed benefit from treatment with* [prolactin] *antagonists in the future.*"

It has also been discovered that higher prolactin readings in men within the normal range are associated with insulin resistance and an imbalance in blood glucose levels.[26] As you will soon see, both of these states are detrimental to the growth of your hair.

How to Avoid Elevated Prolactin

The most consistent stimulus for prolactin secretion in men is stress. To reduce this hormone you need to decrease all forms of stress (see part 6), lower your oestrogen and make sure your thyroid is healthy. Eating foods rich in zinc, vitamin E, vitamin B_6 (such as grass-fed beef, pistachios and avocados) as well as the herbs ashwagandha and mucuna pruriens can be beneficial. Pterostilbene (one of the phytonutrients in blueberries) has also been shown to help.[27]

Cortisol

Produced in the adrenal glands, the primary role of this hormone is to increase blood glucose to provide fuel during a stressful situation. When you encounter a perceived threat, whether real or imaginary, levels of cortisol rise. Once this threat has passed, these should drop and return to normal. Unfortunately, in our current high-stress culture, the body's stress response is activated so often that it doesn't have a chance to return to normal, resulting in a state of chronic stress and elevated cortisol. Prolonged high levels of this hormone are known to affect negatively the function and growth cycle of the hair follicle. Cortisol is yet another enemy of your hair.

In a 2016 study researchers concluded that: "...*excess cortisol is therefore able to exert a disruptive effect on the fine-tuned mechanism of the hair follicle, leading to the development of hair growth disorders such as androgenetic alopecia* [MPB]."[28] Put differently, a continued high level of cortisol makes your hair fall out. This hormone has also been shown to be elevated in men with hair loss. A 1991 study examined sixty-five men suffering from MPB and showed significant differences compared to control subjects.[15]

Prolonged levels of circulating cortisol can cause many problems that negatively affect the growth of your hair including: overproduction of sebum; blood sugar imbalances; sleep disruption; suppression of thyroid hormones; inflammation; decreased liver detoxification of excess oestrogen; calcification of blood vessels; nutritional deficiencies including magnesium, vitamin B_{12} and C and gut inflammation. High cortisol can also stimulate prolactin release and induce activity of the aromatase enzyme[29] leading to elevated oestrogen and lowered testosterone. Oestrogen then stimulates more cortisol production in a vicious cycle. Do not underestimate the power of stress. Chronic stress and elevated cortisol levels are the enemies of a balanced hormonal system.

How to Avoid Elevated Cortisol

Factors that improve cortisol levels include: lowering stress; reducing oestrogen; increasing dietary intakes of magnesium, zinc, omega-3 fatty acids and vitamin C; ashwagandha root; exercise; massage therapy; and enjoying life. Factors that upset cortisol levels include: viral infections, excess caffeine and alcohol, polyunsaturated fatty acids, processed foods, sleep deprivation, excessive exercise, stressful situations and systemic inflammation. If we can reduce inflammation in the body then decreased cortisol levels should follow.

Insulin

This is one of the body's most important hormones. Insulin regulates blood sugar (glucose) and is responsible for allowing this glucose to enter cells, providing them with energy to function. As glucose is one of the main fuels for hair growth, any problems with insulin will mean less energy available for hair follicles, resulting in poorer growth. If insulin levels are either too low or too high, other hormones will be affected adversely and serious health problems such as insulin resistance might start to develop. This is when the cells in your body start resisting or ignoring the signal that this hormone is trying to send out, resulting in elevated blood sugar levels.

Men with insulin resistance are more likely to be bald. A 2005 study found that men with MPB before thirty years of age had significantly higher insulin resistance and greater risk of developing type 2 diabetes.[30] Persistently high blood sugar levels can possibly lead to constriction of blood vessels or damage the vessels themselves. This leads to restriction of blood flow and the supply of oxygen and other nutrients causing a negative impact on the growth of hair follicles.

The idea that just eating too much sugar or refined carbohydrates results in insulin resistance is inaccurate. Although the exact cause of this condition is unknown, several other factors have been linked with insulin resistance. These include: inflammation, obesity and lack of physical activity, chronic stress, food sensitivities, sleep deprivation, prescription and recreational drugs, an unhealthy gut microbiome and diets high in omega-6 polyunsaturated fats (PUFAs).[31]

Metabolic syndrome is the clinical manifestation of insulin resistance and is a dysfunction of energy storage and utilization. Metabolic syndrome isn't a condition in itself but rather a collection of risk factors that can set the stage for type 2 diabetes and heart disease. These risk factors, apart from insulin resistance, include: elevated blood pressure, abnormal cholesterol levels, high triglycerides, vitamin D deficiency and a large waist circumference. A 2013 study conducted on eighty Thai men found that patients with early onset MPB had a 3.48-fold higher risk of metabolic syndrome.[32] A more recent 2018 study on fifty-seven patients with MPB concluded: *"there is significant association between metabolic syndrome and androgenic alopecia."*[33]

Insulin and Circulating Lipids

"The real issue is not baldness having a direct effect on the heart, but that it's a warning of possible heart disease." Dr Gregg Fonarow, professor of cardiovascular medicine at the University of California

Hair loss could be an indication of these metabolic abnormalities as there appears to be a strong association between hair loss, insulin resistance and abnormal levels of circulating lipids (fats). Elevated lipids in the blood, in particular cholesterol and triglycerides, are a major risk factor for cardiovascular disease. Men with MPB show statistically significant abnormal levels of these circulating lipids which might partly explain the association between MPB and cardiovascular disease.

A 2017 review not only found that insulin levels were notably higher in men with early onset MPB but also there were significant differences in circulating lipids.[34] Total cholesterol and triglycerides were higher, whereas HDL cholesterol reflected a trend toward lower levels. *"[T]he results of this meta-analysis support the hypothesis that men with early-onset AGA* [MPB] *are at risk for metabolic impairment, having a worse (although still normal) metabolic profile."* In this review, men with early onset MPB were also found to have higher body mass index values and lower levels of SHBG compared with controls. This represented signs of metabolic syndrome.

An earlier 2014 meta-analysis showed similar results on 154 men aged between nineteen and fifty years with age-matched controls.[35] Only men whose hair loss was significant, using an accepted classification method, were selected. The researchers concluded that: *"Alopecia is associated with an increased risk of coronary heart disease, and there appears to be a dose-response relationship with degree of baldness whereby the greater the severity of alopecia, the greater the risk of coronary heart disease. Alopecia is also associated with an increased risk of hypertension, hyperinsulinaemia, insulin resistance, metabolic syndrome, and having elevated serum total cholesterol and triglyceride levels."* In addition, it was suggested that men with early onset MPB should be screened for insulin resistance and other cardiovascular disease risk factors.

How to Avoid Elevated Insulin and Abnormal Circulating Lipids

Any substance or process that decreases blood glucose levels, improves insulin sensitivity or normalizes circulating lipids is likely to be beneficial for your hair growth. This includes: avoiding PUFAs, artificial sweeteners, fried foods and processed carbohydrates; limiting or eliminating recreational drugs and unnecessary prescription medications; exercising regularly; lowering body mass index and maintaining a healthy weight; testing yourself for any allergies you may have and eliminate that particular food and making sleep a priority. Some foods that may help to decrease insulin levels include: cinnamon, blueberries and other berries, avocado, garlic and other alliums, aloe vera, fermented foods, seaweed, moringa, raw apple cider vinegar and foods containing the phytonutrient myricetin.

Increased inflammation and oxidative stress may contribute to insulin resistance[36,37,38] and there is also some evidence suggesting that an unhealthy gut microbiome[39] could exacerbate this condition. These issues should also be addressed.

A Final Word on Hormones

Several different hormones play a role in hair growth. The idea of blaming a single one on hair loss and ignoring the rest is not only an oversimplification of an extremely complex process but also inaccurate. All of the seven hormones discussed are major players in the growth of the hair follicle. Testosterone, DHT and thyroid hormone are promoters of growth and their production should be encouraged. Oestrogen, prolactin, cortisol and insulin are, however, all inhibitors and their production should be actively reduced.

However, one crucial factor is that these 'negative' hormones have all been shown to lead to an imbalance in blood sugar (glucose). Any process that reduces the delivery of glucose will lead to a disturbance in the energy supply to hair follicles and negatively impact growth. On the contrary, androgens and thyroid hormone are beneficial for hair growth and have positive effects on glucose metabolism.

Another detail to consider is that oestrogen, prolactin, cortisol and insulin are all stimulated by or generate the release of inflammatory chemicals that cause hair loss. These hormones are also related to the stress response and their levels increase in times of stress. Alternately, testosterone, DHT and active thyroid hormone have all been shown to reduce both the release of these inflammatory chemicals and stress levels.

Treating hair loss should be less about targeting a single hormone and more about bringing several hormones into balance, combined with lowering inflammation and stress. As we have seen, these are all factors within your control.

Oxidative Stress and Lipid Peroxidation

Oxidative stress is an imbalance between the production of pro-oxidants (reactive oxygen species [ROS] and free radicals) and their elimination by antioxidants (superoxide dismutase [SOD], vitamins E and C and glutathione). Antioxidants are protective compounds that inhibit oxidation, a chemical reaction that can lead to the damage and destruction of cells. On the other hand, pro-oxidants are compounds that induce oxidation and cause oxidative damage to cells, tissues and organs.

Antioxidants are beneficial for your hair growth while oxidative stress and excess pro-oxidants are detrimental. An excess can be caused by such things as a poor diet, pollution, drugs, toxin exposure and an antioxidant deficiency. As we age, the creation of pro-oxidants increases, while our internal production of anti-oxidants decreases. The resulting increased oxidative stress is one reason why we lose our hair more as we get older.

The presence of oxidative stress in the dermal papilla cells of hair follicles in patients with MPB was confirmed in a 2015 study.[40] The researchers concluded that oxidative stress may be causing hair loss by ageing the cells of the follicles as well as promoting the release of inflammatory chemicals known to inhibit growth. Another 2015 study also revealed that oxidative stress reduced the growth phase of the hair follicle and decreased levels of the antioxidant SOD.[41]

An earlier 2013 study suggested that the release of one of these inflammatory chemicals TGF-beta1 is mediated by the pro-oxidant ROS in the dermal papilla cells.[42] The progression of MPB and inflammation is associated with elevated TGF-beta1. It is also known that ROS levels are increased by inflammation and high blood glucose and reduced by antioxidants. This study concluded:

"...*our findings suggest the potential use of antioxidant therapy for the treatment of androgenic alopecia* [MPB]." Antioxidants can potentially promote hair growth by reducing ROS and subsequently TGF-beta1, a known inhibitor of hair growth.

The increase of DHT in the scalps of men with hair loss could in part be owing to oxidative stress and higher levels of pro-oxidants. Oxidative stress has been shown to increase the entry of DHT into dermal papilla cells while ROS is associated with a higher 5-alpha reductase concentration and activity: consequently, more testosterone is converted to DHT.[43]

Oxidative stress also causes a type of oxidative damage known as lipid peroxidation. This process is where fats in the cell membranes are degraded leading to cell death and the release of inflammatory chemicals like prostaglandins and lipid peroxides. Both of these chemicals are known to cause hair loss. Lipid peroxides are also key mediators in inflammation and cause further generation of ROS, leading to additional oxidative stress.

In a 2008 study researchers concluded that lipid peroxidation may play a role in the development of hair loss.[44] The topical application of lipid peroxides stopped the growth phase in the follicles of mice. Furthermore, they found that lipid peroxides induce death of hair follicle cells and human epidermal (skin) cells.

Lipid peroxidation is associated with the type of fat in the diet. PUFAs are preferentially oxidized while saturated fats in the body generally resist peroxidation.[45] Researchers looked at the impact of dietary oils and fats and concluded: "*The results demonstrated that feeding oils rich in polyunsaturated fatty acids (PUFA) increases lipid peroxidation significantly and may raise the susceptibility of tissues to free radical oxidative damage.*"[46] This means that a diet rich in PUFAs will increase your levels of oxidative stress and chemicals known to cause hair loss.

Inflammation

A certain degree of inflammation is a basic mechanism of a healthy immune system with acute inflammation often serving a protective role. Chronic inflammation, however, leads to tissue destruction and disease. It has been found to be at the root of many disorders and degenerative conditions in the body. The way someone responds to inflammation varies from person to person but as long as whatever is causing the problem is still present, the imbalance remains and continues to harm the body. Early symptoms of chronic inflammation might be vague, with subtle signs and symptoms that may go undetected for a long time. Many of the factors leading to this condition are lifestyle-related. You can control and possibly even reverse chronic inflammation through a healthy anti-inflammatory diet and lifestyle.

A 2009 study studied forty subjects with MPB.[47] The bald area of patients showed highly significant increases in the number of hairs in the resting phase compared to non-balding areas. Tissue inflammation surrounding hair follicles was almost a constant feature in cases of early onset hair loss. Researchers concluded inflammation played an integral role in the development of early onset MPB.

A 2013 study tested a combination of the hair loss drug minoxidil, a nonsteroidal anti-inflammatory agent and tea tree oil (an anti-infective agent).[48] This combination was significantly superior to minoxidil alone in terms of efficacy and achieved an earlier response. These results suggested that both inflammation of the hair follicle and a microbial or fungal infection may be contributing to MPB. The researchers concluded MPB was multi-factorial in nature.

A 1999 study looked at nineteen patients and found significant inflammation around the hair follicles in those with hair loss.[49] *"These data support the idea that the inflammatory process may be, at least in part, responsible for the development of male pattern alopecia."*

An earlier 1991 study looked at twenty-six subjects with hair loss and the researchers confirmed that inflammation is directly involved in the development of MPB.[50]

Men with hair loss have been shown to have enlarged sebaceous glands and increased sebum production. A 1975 study looked at the scalp tissues from twenty-three patients with MPB.[51] The researchers found a marked enlargement of the sebaceous glands: an increased number of mast cells indicating the presence of inflammation as well as fibrosis beneath hair follicles that were shrinking. Sebum exhibits strong antimicrobial activity, transports antioxidants to the skin surface and can express both pro-inflammatory and anti-inflammatory properties.[52] This indicates an increased sebum production could be owing to the presence of oxidative stress and/or inflammation.

Apart from a direct causal role in hair loss, inflammation may be associated with hormonal disturbances. Findings suggest that low testosterone and obesity are both promoters of inflammation.[53] Conversely, the data from 809 men were examined and it was found that higher androgen and lower oestrogen levels may have an anti-inflammatory effect.[54] Inflammation is also associated with lipid peroxidation and oxidative stress. In a 2017 review researchers stated that: *"A growing body of work implicates lipid peroxides as key mediators of many pathological states including inflammation."*[55] The generation of the pro-oxidant ROS also brings about inflammation, whilst in a vicious cycle, inflammation causes further production of ROS.

Therefore, there is considerable evidence showing inflammation is involved with MPB, though this is not always obvious or visible to the eye. This idea explains why prematurely bald men are also more likely to suffer from other problems such as diabetes, obesity and heart disease. All of these conditions are linked to chronic inflammation.

How to Avoid Oxidative Stress, Lipid Peroxidation and Inflammation

Dietary improvements will probably have the greatest impact overall on reducing oxidative stress, lipid peroxidation and inflammation. The foods that cause these imbalances are not found in abundance in nature. The modern diet, however, most certainly is a generous source though the problems associated with poor food choices can initially occur without obvious symptoms. Even so, over time a diet rich in processed foods, refined grains and PUFAs lead to the chronic diseases that plague modern man, including hair loss.

On the other hand, an excellent diet provides your body with all of the antioxidants it needs. Vitamins A and D both play a major role in the control of the inflammatory response. Vitamins C and E, as well as selenium, zinc, glutathione and melatonin are powerful antioxidants. Thyroid hormones can have a protective role against oxidative damage, so iodine and iron are also important.[56]

Turmeric root, cardamom and the herb mucuna pruriens have been shown to be useful in lowering level of lipid peroxidation. You can also reduce your exposure to fluoride and toxic metals such as cadmium (see part 6) which are known to increase levels.

Although it may seem a lot easier to reduce inflammation by going to your local drug store, there are problems with this approach. Nonsteroidal anti-inflammatory drugs (NSAIDs) such as aspirin, ibuprofen and naproxen all come with undesirable reactions like: stomach bleeding, damage of the gut lining, fewer numbers of good bacteria in your gut,[57] an increased potential of liver and kidney disease and heart attacks. Many allergy medications work as antihistamines that reduce inflammation. Histamine blocking agents are unsuitable for long-term use as they can, among other effects, cause breast enlargement in men and a decrease in sperm count.

Apart from dietary considerations, there are also many environmental and lifestyle factors that lead to oxidative stress and chronic inflammation including: the use of prescription and recreational drugs; exposure to synthetic xenoestrogens, toxic heavy metals and other chemical pollutants; allergens like mould; cigarette smoke; dehydration; lack of and excessive exercise; deficient sleep and poorly functioning liver, thyroid and digestive system.

Getting Tested for Cortisol, Prolactin, Insulin, Stress and Inflammation

Cortisol/DHEA-S Saliva Test: This measures the levels of the stress hormones DHEA-S and cortisol to help evaluate adrenal function. The preferred method tests four salivary samples and provides an evaluation of how these levels differ throughout the day.

hs-CRP (not the standard CRP test): Measures C-reactive protein (CRP), a protein that increases in the blood with inflammation. Apart from acute infection/injury, CRP is also an indicator of chronic inflammation. Optimal CRP levels to strive for are under 0.55 mg/L.

Prolactin: The upper threshold of normal prolactin is about 20 µg/L (425 mIU/L). Ideal levels for men are between 5-10 µg/L. Prolactin strongly indicates oestrogen dominance if it is high. An elevated reading also indicates the thyroid gland is underactive and there are possibly problems with the adrenals.

There is no one test that can directly detect insulin resistance. Laboratory tests most likely to be ordered include:

Fasting plasma glucose (FPG): This is usually performed fasting and determines an impaired response to glucose. A level between 70 and 100 mg/dL is considered normal; above this, your body is showing signs of insulin resistance and diabetes. Ideally, you want to have a reading of less than 85 mg/dL.

Fasting insulin: You want this reading to be ideally below 5 uIU/mL. A high level of fasting insulin indicates insulin resistance and metabolic syndrome.

Fasting cholesterol (total triglycerides, HDL and LDL): Total cholesterol should be less than 150 mg/dL. Normal triglyceride levels are less than 150 mg/dL (ideally under 100 mg/dL). An optimal level of HDL cholesterol should be between 55-150 mg/dL. LDL cholesterol should be between 80-120 mg/dL. Insulin resistance and hair loss are both associated with increases in total cholesterol, triglycerides, and LDL as well as a decrease in HDL. Elevated cholesterol may indicate a problem with the thyroid.

Hair Growth Modulators

Several hundred modulators (regulators) involved in hair growth have been identified. Recognised inhibitory factors include TGF-beta1, FGF-5 and mast cells which release prostaglandins and cytokines (such as TNF). All of these chemicals have been shown to be increased in the scalps of men with MPB. They are inhibitors of the growth phase of hair follicles as well as being part of the inflammatory process.

Prostaglandin D_2 (PGD$_2$): The prostaglandins are a group of lipids made at sites of tissue damage and play a key role in the generation of the inflammatory response. Their synthesis is significantly increased in inflamed tissue, whether acute or chronic. Any process that increases the levels of chronic inflammation will result in the release of PGD$_2$. Prostaglandins are also significantly involved in calcification and fibrosis[58] (see the next section).

A 2012 study discovered a link between PGD$_2$ elevation and hair loss, first in mice and then in men.[59] They demonstrated that PGD$_2$ was elevated in balding areas (but not in hair-bearing areas) of men with MPB. This prostaglandin has the capacity to decrease hair lengthening and cause hair loss.

In a 2018 study researchers concluded that PGD$_2$ (not just DHT) could be involved in the activation of androgen receptors.[60] According to the androgen theory, activation of these receptors in dermal papilla cells is regarded as the beginning of hair miniaturization and eventual hair loss. The study showed chronic inflammation and the release of PGD_2 was responsible for this initial activation. Chronic inflammation not DHT, therefore, could be the starting point of hair loss.

To reduce the release of this chemical, you need to decrease levels of inflammation and lipid peroxidation. Known inhibitors of PGD_2 and other inflammatory prostaglandins include: ginger root, ricinoleic acid (found in castor oil), aloe vera, foods rich in manganese such as cardamom and cloves, and various phytonutrients including salicin, luteolin, apeginin, quercetin and resveratrol.

Transforming Growth Factor beta 1(TGF-beta1): This is a growth factor vital in several biological processes including inflammation, fibrosis and calcification.[61] TGF-beta1 levels are related to the progression of MPB and increased levels of prostaglandins. It is part of an inflammation response that reduces nutrient supply to the hair follicles and leads to fewer hairs in the growth phase.

A 2000 study found that injecting TGF-beta1 into mice stopped the growth phase of hair follicles.[62] This modulator also increases ROS production and suppresses antioxidants, leading to oxidative stress. ROS, in turn, activates TGF-beta1, forming a vicious cycle.[63] The hair loss drug finasteride has been shown to lower levels of this modulator, which may in part explain some of its efficacy.[64]

PUFAs, low thyroid function, excess oestrogen, zinc deficiency, stress and toxic mould exposure all lead to an increase in levels. Foods known to decrease TGF-beta1 include: turmeric, olives and olive oil, sea vegetables, aloe vera, the herbs He shou wu and milk thistle, as well as various phytonutrients including apigenin, quercetin and narigenin.

Tumor Necrosis Factor (TNF): This is a pro-inflammatory chemical messenger that can lead to cell death in the hair bulb. A 1996 study found that TNF was a potent inhibitor of hair follicle growth.[65] A later 2019 study stated that a low testosterone level is correlated with increased expression of this modulator and other markers of inflammation.[66] TNF also adversely affects thyroid function[67] and the digestive system.

TNF is increased by sleep deprivation; high blood glucose levels;[68] lack of and too much exercise; infections; stress; obesity;

excess alcohol consumption; heavy metal toxicity; smoking; as well as deficiencies in vitamin D, magnesium and zinc. Both testosterone[69] and DHT[70] have been shown to *inhibit* TNF. The South American herb cat's claw is a potent inhibitor of its production as well as: nettle leaf, ashwagandha, cinnamon, turmeric, boswellia, horny goat weed, horsetail, cardamom, white willow bark and the phytonutrient resveratrol.

Fibroblast Growth Factor 5 (FGF-5): Blocking this modulator in the human scalp results in less hair fall and increased growth. A 2002 study showed that FGF-5 reduces hair growth by stopping the growth phase and blocking dermal papilla cell activation.[71] The herbs great burnet and rosemary, citrus fruits and eucalyptus are all known inhibitors.

As we can see, several modulators have been revealed in various studies to affect negatively hair growth. The fact that these modulators are all mediators of inflammation reinforces the concept that these two processes are connected. There is also evidence showing that inflammatory chemicals could be initiating the hair loss process. Rather than looking for the next drug or treatment, the effects of these modulators can be decreased naturally. Various foods and herbs as well as lifestyle changes are all proven ways to do just this.

Fibrosis and Calcification

The final factor to consider is that any process that limits the availability of oxygen and other nutrients to the scalp and follicles will impede hair growth. A lack of oxygen (hypoxia) in follicles as well as a reduction in blood flow has been shown in the balding areas of men with MPB. One theory by which the popular drug minoxidil (Rogaine or Regaine) works is it widens blood vessels and so allows more oxygen and nutrients to the follicles.[72] This will then lead to thicker and healthier hair.

In one small 1996 study it was shown that men's balding regions had just 60 percent of the oxygen levels of non-balding areas.[73] Men with no hair loss had oxygen levels nearly the same all across their scalp.

In an earlier 1989 study researchers measured the subcutaneous blood flow in the scalps of those with and without hair loss.[74] In men with early onset MPB the blood flow was over two and a half times lower than the values found in controls. They concluded that: "*A reduced nutritive blood flow to the hair follicles might be a significant event in the pathogenesis* [development] *of early male pattern baldness.*"

In a 2010 study forty men aged between nineteen and fifty-seven with MPB were tested.[75] Each subject was injected with botox (botulinum toxin) in over thirty sites on their scalp over a period of sixty weeks. The researchers reported obvious hair regrowth in several subjects. They concluded that botox increases blood flow and oxygen concentration to the scalp. "*Blood flow may therefore be a primary determinant in follicular health.*"

In a similar more recent 2017 study, ten men were injected in thirty sites with botox; and the process repeated twenty-four weeks later.[76] Eight of the men had a good to excellent response. The researchers found that these intramuscular injections relaxed the muscles in the scalp and thereby potentially elevated both blood and oxygen supply. They hypothesized that the elevated blood flow could reduce DHT levels in the scalp as the conversion from testosterone happens primarily in a low oxygen environment. Increasing blood supply to the scalp could therefore reduce DHT levels.

One reason for this reduction in blood and oxygen could be owing to a process known as fibrosis. Studies have shown that men with MPB not only have significant inflammation in the scalp but also fibrosis surrounding their hair follicles. This happens when excess fibrous connective tissue such as collagen develops and thickens owing to some kind of damage. The process doesn't just occur in response to an obvious injury such as a cut but also happens as a result of chronic inflammation. When it takes place on the scalp, the fibrotic tissue will negatively affect the growth of hair. Fibrosis imposes physical constrictions by lessening the width of follicles which over time leads to a decrease in blood flow and oxygen. This restricted growth space will ultimately cause hair loss and fibrosis appears to develop concurrently with MPB. The most well-known mediator of this process is the inflammatory chemical TGF-beta1[77] but other chemicals such as PGD_2 are involved.

A 2009 study looked at forty patients with MPB.[46] Fibrosis surrounding hair follicles was more marked in advanced cases of hair loss and the researchers concluded that fibrosis sometimes causes complete destruction of the affected follicles.

In an earlier 2008 study ten men aged twenty to thirty-five with MPB were found to have a near four-fold increase in collagen fibres (fibrosis) on their scalps, compared with controls.[78] The total number of mast cells was also about two-fold higher than normal, indicating the presence of inflammation.

A small 1992 study found measurable fibrosis in the scalps of patients with MPB.[79] They also found mast cell degranulation in the hair follicles. This process involves the release of various inflammatory substances including PGD_2. A deficiency of oxygen is known to increase the concentration of mast cells within a tissue.

Another possible reason for the reduction in oxygen and blood flow to the scalp could be calcification. This is the build-up of calcium in body tissue and other places. These hard deposits are found in tissues chronically inflamed and the chemicals PGD_2 and TGF-beta1 both stimulate this process.[58,62] These calcium deposits are known to accumulate in the inflamed tissue of the scalp as well as the blood vessels that supply the scalp.

Back in 1942 Dr Frederick Hoelzel published the connection between calcification, restricted blood flow and hair loss.[80] When removing the brains of cadavers, he discovered calcification in some of the men with hair loss. It was severe enough not only to fuse together the fibrous connective tissue between adjacent bones of the skull but also to close completely the narrow openings through which blood vessels and nerves pass. These blood vessels are the ones providing the hair follicles with nutrients and oxygen. If the nerve supply is blocked, this would explain why bald areas are less sensitive than non-bald areas of the scalp. Men with no signs of hair loss did not have this problem with calcification and reduced blood supply.

A recent 2019 study found an increased risk of heart disease in men with hair loss.[81] The researchers concluded the associations between heart disease and MPB may be driven by the cumulative effect of shared factors connecting the two conditions: diabetes, increased body mass index and calcium deposits in the coronary arteries. Calcification happens in any inflamed tissue of the body whether the scalp or an artery.

Hypertension (high blood pressure) and MPB have also been found to be significantly associated with each other.[82] Researchers are unsure of the reasons behind the connection, but it's possible hypertension restricts blood supply to the hair follicles. Minoxidil was first introduced as medication for elevated blood pressure before the development of a topical formulation for promoting hair growth. One theory is that this drug works by relaxing muscles in the walls of blood vessels. This then reduces blood pressure and allows an increase in circulating nutrients and oxygen.

How to Avoid Fibrosis and Calcification

Any process, whether high blood pressure, fibrosis or calcification that restricts blood flow to the scalp will be detrimental to hair growth leading to slow but eventual loss. Techniques that improve circulation to the scalp such as massage and inverted postures will be helpful. However, low oxygen availability and reduced blood flow are symptoms and not direct causes of hair loss. Managing these symptoms will certainly help by reversing some of the damage that has been done but at the same time you should also be treating the causes.

Anything that negatively affects thyroid health will reduce the quantity of oxygen and other nutrients such as glucose being delivered to the hair follicles. So thyroid function needs to be addressed. As fibrosis appears to be mediated by TGF-beta1 and other inflammatory chemicals like PGD_2, you need to focus on reducing overall levels of inflammation as well.

The blood vessels that support the follicles become calcified when there is too much calcium present in the bloodstream. This excess can be caused by: too much phosphate in the diet; fluorine intake or exposure;[83] lowered thyroid hormones;[84] high cortisol levels; calcium and vitamin D supplements; deficiencies in calcium, magnesium[85] and the vitamins D and K_2. It is extremely important to have the correct balance of calcium and magnesium in the body to prevent calcification.

What Does All This Mean?

MPB is a chronic condition. It is an issue that comes over time, usually many years, and yet we tend to view and treat it as an acute problem. As with other chronic conditions different factors, often working in tandem, lead to the same symptom. The underlying reason for your hair loss is probably a combination of both inflammation and oxidative stress. These are closely related processes, one can be easily induced by the other and both are found in many pathological conditions. Several different imbalances can all produce the same symptom: hair loss. As the actual cause of MPB may vary greatly from person to person, there can't be a single diagnosis or cure. A variety of treatments must apply. An individual cause or single hormone cannot be isolated and held responsible for hair loss in all men.

Medication is not your only option. A natural solution is desirable as this will resolve any underlying issues and give you more permanent results. The rest of this book can help you address the underlying causes of hair loss and not just the symptoms. Obviously some of these changes will make a greater impact than others. However, they take time to achieve. Your hair loss didn't occur in one day so don't expect to fix it overnight either.

Part 3: Nutrients and Body Systems

"Fast food and junk food, preservatives and additives, chemically contaminated air and water, mad-dash lifestyles and indiscriminate use of drugs, both medical and recreational, have all contributed to the overall degradation of human health and the relentless pollution of the human body." Daniel P. Reid, *The Tao of Detox*

The single most effective and realistic approach to transforming the health of your hair is to start eating better. It is well documented that type 2 diabetes, heart disease, cancers and other inflammatory diseases are all directly the result of a poor diet. Why does the idea that hair loss could also be the result of this unnatural way of eating seem so strange? Specific foods and herbs are known to decrease inflammation and the activity of inhibitory hair growth modulators. Antioxidants have been shown to lower oxidative stress and lipid peroxidation, as well as improving glucose metabolism. Nutritional imbalances increase oestrogen, cortisol and insulin as well as decreasing testosterone and active thyroid hormone. Imbalances also lead to calcification and severe deficiencies can directly lead to hair loss. This all shows that correct nutritional balance is clearly essential not just for your general health but also for optimal hair growth.

We can't focus on hair specifically without taking the overall condition of our body into account. There is no separation between the health of your body and that of your hair. If you are experiencing any health problems or suffering from nutritional deficiencies, your hair may stop growing or show damage. Our hair is part of, not separate from, our body. Poor nutrition is an extremely crucial factor in explaining MPB but it is by no means the only offender. Many men are sceptical about the efficacy of natural foods for preventing their problem. I agree that minor changes to your diet don't make much difference, especially over the short-term. The more diverse your diet, the better. However, no one single food, vitamin, spice or herb will cure your hair loss. There is no magic nutritional bullet or Holy Grail.

There is also no single ideal human diet as we are adapted to a wide range of diverse foods. We have distinct needs and tastes, different bodies and individual lives. Our dietary needs vary according to many factors including age, body type, metabolic rate, level of activity, medications, allergies and general overall health. Our culinary desires and personal tastes differ as well as what is found in our local shops, the climate and what we can afford. This all makes for a single nutritional approach unrealistic. However, certain foods are definitely best avoided while others are highly recommended for healthy hair.

Not Getting Enough? Common Nutritional Deficiencies

"About one-half of American adults have one or more preventable, chronic disease related to suboptimal diet and physical activity patterns, and more than two-thirds of adults are overweight or obese." 2015 Dietary Guidelines Advisory Committee

In a 2009 article the authors reviewed the National Health and Nutrition Examination Survey from 2003-2004.[1] US recommendations aim for a feasible rather than an optimal intake: two to three cups vegetables and one and a half to two servings of fruit a day. Around 2 percent of men in the US met these recommendations, despite this figure including jam, jelly, orange juice, French fries and ketchup. Orange juice was the main fruit choice and potatoes the dominant vegetable.

Inadequate dietary intakes of vitamins, minerals and phytonutrients are common even in countries that have traditionally eaten lots of fresh fruits and vegetables. This can happen because of an energy-rich, nutrient-poor and processed diet. In addition, excessive use of alcohol and drugs, together with elevated stress can further deplete levels. Whether you realise it or not, you are probably lacking or suboptimal in at least one essential nutrient. Get tested and then direct your efforts to specifically target any problems.

It may not be enough to have levels that are in the 'reference range'. These ranges are mathematically calculated from the average readings of a large population; they are not an indication of ideal levels. Nora T. Gedgaudas says this in her book *Primal Body, Primal Mind*: *"As the population gets less and less healthy and everything gets averaged out, many lab ranges have become too broad to be meaningful to a major portion of the population. They don't tell you in the least how you compare with 'normal and healthy.' The lab ranges are exclusively meant to reveal pathologic conditions, which may or may not be accurately represented."*

Try getting your readings of all essential vitamins and minerals toward the high end. Levels that are not optimal, even if within the normal range, may not be enough to ensure ideal hair growth especially as individual requirements vary widely. A few studies show the extent of common nutrient deficiencies even within these wide reference ranges.

Ten men were tested, both athletes and sedentary people, and were found to have at least two or more nutrient deficiencies.[2] Their diets were found to be lacking in: iodine (100 percent), vitamin D (90 percent), zinc and vitamin E (both 80 percent), selenium (70 percent), magnesium (60 percent), calcium and vitamins B_6 and K_1 (all 50 percent), vitamins A and B_2 (both 30 percent), vitamins B_1, B_3 and B_9 (all 20 percent) and vitamin B_{12} (10 percent).

The 2011 *National Health and Nutrition Examination Survey* showed that the deficiencies in American adults were: vitamin D (95 percent), vitamin E (94 percent), magnesium (61 percent), vitamin A (51 percent), calcium (49 percent), vitamin C (43 percent), vitamin B_6 (15 percent), vitamin B_9 (13 percent), zinc (12 percent) and iron (8 percent).[3]

Certain nutritional deficiencies are known to be associated with hair loss. Some studies are starting to show more precise data:

•A 2017 study looked at thirty-four men with MPB.[4] They were found to be deficient in various nutrients including: nineteen in the amino acid cysteine, thirty-one in vitamin B_9 (folate), three in vitamin B_{12}, three in vitamin B_7 (biotin), four in zinc, ten in copper and four in ferritin (stored iron).

•A 2013 study assessed patients with different types of hair loss and found that serum zinc levels were lower in all hair loss patients compared to controls.[5] Several with MPB had extremely low zinc levels.

•A 1998 study evaluated the zinc, copper, iron and manganese status of men with MPB compared to controls.[6] The zinc and manganese levels were significantly lower while copper levels were significantly higher in men with MPB. There was no statistical difference in the iron levels between the two groups.

All of these studies support the idea that you should test yourself for any deficiencies, then do your best to correct them, as they could be an obvious part of the problem. If you are lacking in any nutrient, you may not be getting enough in your diet or there might be an underlying issue. For example, zinc deficiency can be caused by various factors and not only reduced dietary intake. Inadequate absorption of this mineral could be from an underactive thyroid, problems with acidity levels of the stomach or excessive consumption of phytic acid. Increased loss could be from exercise, high alcohol intake or medications. The answer may not necessarily be as simple as getting more in your food or taking a supplement. Other issues possibly need to be addressed.

Supplements

"Bottom line, getting well is about healthy eating and detoxifying, not taking medicine or vitamin pills." Donna Gates, The Body Ecology Diet

Many people are now taking supplements on top of a normal diet. In recent times, supplementing has shifted from trying to prevent deficiencies to taking higher amounts of various vitamins and minerals in an effort to enhance health. As Catherine Price says in her book *Vitamania*: *"…we use vitamins as insurance policies against whatever else we might (or might not) be eating, as if by atoning for our other nutritional sins, vitamins can save us from ourselves. We think that vitamins will help us live longer and stay healthier, even prevent or reverse disease."*

When it comes to obtaining nutrients, your diet and not supplements should be your primary source. You will be missing out on all the other chemicals that naturally exist in foods that are not present in multivitamins. If you are eating junk food then your nutritional needs will not be met by taking a pill: you cannot supplement your way out of a poor diet. There is no reason to take a daily multivitamin 'just in case' if eating well. Nutrients should come from food, not from a laboratory. Supplements may be doing people who eat a healthy diet more harm than good as they can interfere with nutrient absorption or cause other side effects.

In the words of author Sandor Ellis Katz from his book *The Revolution Will Not be Microwaved*: *"Fortified, reconstituted food products are regarded as the equivalent of fresh, nutritious whole foods. Synthetic nutrient encapsulation in the form of supplements is another presumed equivalent. The idea that synthetic powders in a capsule could really give us everything that food does is a delusion."*

A product made with isolated compounds is not necessarily safe, especially if these are hundreds or thousands of times more concentrated than found in nature. Scientific studies have consistently shown vitamin supplements don't prevent disease or improve health. In some cases, they might increase your risk of cardiovascular disease, cancer and mortality. In 2017 the *Journal of Nutrition and Food Sciences* came to this conclusion: *"Inappropriate combinations and nutrient overdose are easily possible with rising use of multivitamins and fortified foods."*[7]

Even natural vitamin supplements can be mostly synthetic. When a vitamin is marked 'natural,' it only has to include 10 percent of actual plant-derived ingredients. The other 90 percent could be from synthetic sources like coal tar, acetone or formaldehyde. If you wish to check any product: www.consumerlab.com is a useful resource. It independently tests health and nutritional products randomly chosen from store shelves and verifies their ingredients.

High intakes of antioxidants (vitamins A, E, C and beta-carotene) have been shown to reverse their benefits and behave as pro-oxidants.[8] In other words; these vitamins in supplement form can induce oxidative stress, subsequently increase inflammation and contribute to your hair loss. A 2017 review showed that over-supplementation of certain nutrients including selenium, vitamin A and vitamin E, has been directly linked to hair loss.[9] It also showed that too much iron can lead to a reduction in testosterone. Another study demonstrated that both calcium and vitamin D as a supplement can cause calcification of blood vessels.[10]

Still, around 50 percent of people in the US and the UK regularly take vitamin supplements. If you are taking a supplement in addition to eating well, you may be reaching vitamin and mineral levels much higher than recommended and causing imbalances. Many multivitamin formulas contain selenium, vitamins A and E, calcium and iron, so they may be directly contributing to your hair loss. Unless you have been told by your doctor to do otherwise, I would focus on getting all your vitamins and minerals from the highest-quality food and unadulterated fresh herbs, and not from a pill bottle. Nature knows best. This should be your goal although this may not always be feasible. Some ongoing supplementation for optimal health may be necessary, especially if you are vitamin D, B_{12} or K_2 deficient: but choose wisely and know they are not the best or natural way to obtain the nutrients your body needs.

Loss of Nutritive Value and Organic Food

Food today is grown to improve traits such as size, growth rate and resistance to pests, but not nutritional content. Our current food industry is based on economics. Quality is far less important than profit.

Researchers studied US Department of Agriculture nutritional data from both 1950 and 1999 for forty-three different vegetables and fruits.[11] They found reliable declines in the amount of protein, calcium, phosphorus, iron and the vitamins B_2 and C over the past half century. The researchers also said that there are likely to have been declines in other nutrients such as magnesium, zinc and vitamins B_6 and E, but they were not studied in 1950. Similar results have been found for produce grown in the UK.[12]

One obvious reason for this is that modern intensive agricultural practices have stripped increasing amounts of nutrients from the soil. Other reasons include the use of pesticides and fertilizers, fast-growing crops, over-cultivation, changing storage and ripening systems as well as different varieties of plants now being grown.

In the further words of Sandor Ellis Katz: *"The same erroneous assumption of equivalence underlies chemical fertilization of the soil. If a chemical additive contains the essential plant nutrients of nitrogen, phosphorous, and potassium in appropriate proportions, then it is assumed to be the equivalent of feeding the soil manure and leaves and kitchen scraps. It just isn't so. The soil is alive and our bodies are alive and these complex life processes require a huge variety of micronutrients in order to thrive. They cannot properly sustain themselves on the limited nutrients provided by synthetic chemicals."*

The term 'organic' refers to the way agricultural products are grown and processed. While the regulations vary between countries, generally organic crops must be grown without the use of synthetic pesticides, bioengineered genes or petroleum-based fertilizers.

Livestock raised for meat, eggs and dairy products must have access to the outdoors and be given organic feed. They may not be given antibiotics (unless necessary), growth hormones or any animal by-products.

Organic food is not a trend. All of humanity ate organic until the early part of the twentieth century. Commercially grown foods may sometimes look better but the quality and nutritive value (as well as taste) is usually inferior.

One review of forty-one scientific studies found that organic crops contained significantly more magnesium, vitamin C, iron, calcium, copper, manganese and protein of higher quality.[13] In another review researchers carried out meta-analyses based on 343 publications and concluded that: *"organic crops, on average, have higher concentrations of antioxidants, lower concentrations of cadmium and a lower incidence of pesticide residues than the non-organic comparators across regions and production seasons."*[14]

One of the reasons for this is that organic soil generally has a higher mineral content than traditional farming soil. Conventional fertilizers are 'simple' chemical compounds which supply very few nutrients and are often contaminated with cadmium. Plants grown in these depleted soils absorb toxic heavy metals such as mercury and arsenic more easily. Eating organic food does not necessarily reduce your intake of these metals though it probably does.

Many common pesticides including glyphosate have been demonstrated to interfere with the endocrine system and raise oestrogen levels. The herbicide atrazine has been banned by the European Union since 2004. In the US it's the second most used pesticide. It is a potent xenoestrogen and researchers have revealed that: *"The popular herbicide atrazine is an endocrine disruptor that demasculinizes and feminizes several species of animals, and co-relates with breast and reproductive disorders in mammalians. We recently reported that atrazine induces human aromatase gene expression."*[15] Both glyphosate and atrazine are banned in organic farming.

Despite general belief, organic farms do use pesticides though your exposure to harmful ones will be considerably lower when eating organic. Some varieties of conventionally grown produce are much higher in pesticide residues than others, whilst others are low enough that buying non-organic is relatively safe. *The Environmental Working Group* (www.ewg.org) offers an annually updated list of what produce is the most and the least contaminated.

Foods that are most consistently contaminated include: strawberries, spinach, nectarines, apples, grapes, peaches, cherries, pears, tomatoes, celery, potatoes, bell peppers, cucumbers, kale, spring greens and chili peppers. Whenever we eat conventionally grown produce, invariably traces of these chemicals are present. We are assured that there are no adverse health effects due to low-level exposure of these residues. Despite restrictions on the amount of each pesticide allowed on a single item, there is no limit to the total number of different pesticides that can be on all of your food.

Animal foods tend to contain more toxic residues than plant foods as they are higher up the food chain. Livestock used for conventional meat and dairy are commonly supplemented with synthetic growth hormones including oestrogen. 70 percent of antibiotics made in the US are given to livestock not just because these animals are raised unnaturally and are vulnerable to disease and infection but primarily as growth promoters. However, organically raised animals must be given organic feed and kept free of growth hormones and antibiotics as much as possible.

Local farmers' markets are generally great places to source organic, seasonal and local food. You can also try growing your own. If you can't buy organic, at least give your produce a decent wash before eating. You can make a safe home-made wash by mixing one part salt with nine parts water. Let the produce soak for ten minutes in a bowl or a sink and rinse well afterward. Some pesticides are found on the surface of foods while others may be taken up through the roots and into the plant and cannot be removed by washing. It's actually a good idea to give both organic and non-organic produces a wash.

More information on organic food can be found at www.soilassociation.org.

Top Hair Nutrients
"The food you eat can be either the safest and most powerful form of medicine or the slowest form of poison." Anne Wigmore

Chronic malnourishment is associated with hair loss but for a nutrient deficiency to cause an obvious problem, this needs to be severe. Diets in the Western world are far from ideal but they usually provide enough nourishment to avoid any extreme deficiencies. Despite that, many men are still chronically lacking or have suboptimal levels in vital nutrients that are important for healthy hair. It is also important to note that vitamins and minerals do not exist or function in isolation. Nutrients are synergistic and these critical interactions between different ones need to be considered. Vitamins A, D and K_2, magnesium and calcium, for example, all work in tandem with each other. If one is lacking, it will affect one or more of the others.

Zinc

Inadequate levels are common in the Western diet. This mineral cannot be stored in the body and many men who suffer from hair loss have been found to have deficiencies. This mineral is important for normal sebum gland function, inhibiting the production of prolactin[16] and regulating thyroid hormones.[17]

Zinc is also extremely important for the production of androgens. When normal young men had their dietary levels restricted for twenty weeks, their testosterone dropped dramatically to just over a quarter of starting levels.[18] Alternately, when older men who were deficient in zinc took supplements for six months, they almost doubled their testosterone levels. One key function of this mineral is reducing the activity of the aromatase enzyme, and so less testosterone is converted to oestrogen.[19]

There are many reasons men are deficient: mineral depleted soils, medications, stress (which can more than triple your rate of zinc excretion), illness, gluten intolerance, phytic acid, alcohol, marijuana, excessive ejaculation (semen has a high concentration of zinc) and exposure to lead, cadmium or mercury. If your body cannot get enough zinc, it will start using selenium instead, possibly leading to a deficiency in this mineral as well. Zinc's absorption is greatly compromised when your stomach acid levels are low. In a potential vicious cycle, zinc is a key nutrient to help make the conditions in the stomach sufficiently acidic.

If you're a vegetarian or vegan, you need to be particularly careful about getting this mineral into your diet. Good sources include: grass-fed lamb, liver, oysters, cacao, green leafy vegetables and raw pumpkin and hemp seeds. To increase the bioavailability of zinc in your food you should soak all nuts, seeds, grains and beans. The Chinese herb He shou wu and burdock root are other sources.

The minerals zinc and copper complement each other so when the levels of one rise, the levels of the other tend to fall. To bring your zinc/copper ratio into balance, it's better to focus on replenishing zinc than reducing copper. Reducing stress, removing any amalgam (mercury) dental fillings, eating foods rich in manganese such as cardamom and cloves and eating organic will all help. Another reason not to take a multivitamin is that it may contain copper which can upset this balance.

Iodine

This is the only mineral that comes from the sea. If you have inadequate iodine, you will not make enough active thyroid hormone which is essential for the development and maintenance of the hair follicle. Single and multiple deficiencies of iodine, selenium and zinc have been shown to have negative effects on thyroid metabolism and structure and, therefore, hair growth.[20]

Iodine deficiency is common in both the US and Europe. Thyroid disorders, which may occur owing to a lack of this mineral, are a common cause of hair loss. A deficiency can result from a lack of iodine-rich foods or food grown on deficient soil. The concentration in soil varies considerably by region with coastal areas having higher levels owing to absorption from the atmosphere. The best source of iodine is sea vegetables. Another good source is wild fish such as sardines, anchovies and haddock.

Fluorine, chlorine and bromine are all chemically similar to iodine. These three chemicals are not only toxic but also are now frequently added to our water, foods and household products. The higher the exposure to these chemicals and the lower your iodine levels, the more likely it is that your thyroid will absorb and store them in place of iodine, effectively displacing this essential nutrient. So, as well as increasing your dietary intake, it is strongly recommended to reduce your exposure to these other three toxic chemicals (see part 6).

Magnesium

Researchers looked at this essential nutrient in the Western diet and concluded that: *"Among US adults, 68 percent consumed less than the recommended daily allowance (RDA) of magnesium, and 19 percent consumed less than 50 percent of the RDA."*[21]

Magnesium has been shown to effectively prevent calcification of blood vessels as it regulates calcium balance.[22] A diet high in calcium and/or phosphorus and low in magnesium is associated with calcification of the scalp and blood vessels.[23,24]

Men who have elevated levels of magnesium tend to have higher free testosterone. In one study, thirty men aged eighteen to twenty-two received ten mg/kg magnesium for four weeks.[25] Their levels of both free and total testosterone increased. The men who were the most active saw the greater increases.

This mineral has been proven to decrease inflammation. The dietary intake was found to be significantly and inversely associated with serum CRP (C-reactive protein) levels.[26] CRP is the standard blood test for low grade or chronic inflammation. Magnesium deficiency has also been shown to increase insulin resistance. In addition, this mineral is critical for the production of the antioxidant glutathione as well as making melatonin and promoting healthy sleep.

The causes of magnesium deficiency vary from inadequate dietary intake to excessive loss from the body. Some causes of this loss include: a diet high in processed food, calcium and iron supplements, low stomach acid, medications such as antibiotics, fluoride exposure, excess alcohol and chronic stress.

There are many foods considered rich in magnesium but, because our soils are becoming depleted, we're not getting as much of this important mineral that we need, particularly from conventionally farmed foods. Excellent sources of magnesium include: sea vegetables, green leafy vegetables especially dandelion greens, cacao beans and shells, pumpkin seeds, figs, walnuts and almonds.

Calcium

This is the most abundant mineral in the human body and essential for proper thyroid function. Having the correct balance of calcium, magnesium, phosphorus and the vitamins D and K_2 is important to prevent calcification. Calcium and phosphorus (phosphate) work on a see-saw effect: when one is up, the other is down. So, we want to increase our calcium intake while decreasing our phosphate consumption. High phosphate foods that should be avoided include: soda/fizzy drinks (especially dark colas), processed dairy and meat products, most fast foods, processed foods in general as well as commercial baked goods.

"The evidence of increasing phosphorus intake is clear, with more compounds being added to the food supply and more foods consumed as processed or pre-prepared, and the risk of exceeding the current upper intake level is feasible for large segments of the population."[27] Just from phosphate additives alone, not including that from natural sources, many people are consuming far too much. Researchers have also found a high normal level of phosphate in the blood is linked to calcification, even in healthy young men.[28]

Parathyroid hormone (PTH) is secreted from four parathyroid glands located behind the thyroid gland. The function of PTH is to manage calcium levels within the blood. If your diet is low in this mineral (or high in phosphate) then PTH will increase the level of calcium in your blood. It achieves this by facilitating removal from skeletal tissues: eventually leading to calcification of the scalp tissue and blood vessels supplying the hair follicles. More calcium and less phosphate in your diet will cause a reduction in PTH to be secreted and subsequently less calcification. PTH also increases prolactin levels and vice versa.

Raw milk, sardines, sea vegetables and green leafy vegetables are all good dietary sources of calcium. On the other hand, high phosphate foods, high protein diets, unfermented soy, PUFAs, excess alcohol, lack of exercise, aluminium containing antacids, antibiotics and vitamin A supplements can all induce a calcium loss. Do not take as a supplement as this can cause calcification and interrupt your magnesium balance.[10]

Iron

A shortage, with or without anaemia, has been linked to hair loss. Iron is one of the most common deficiencies in the world and usually occurs if your diet lacks iron-rich foods or you aren't absorbing it correctly. However, loss of blood and illness can also be a cause. Iron deficiency is often seen with an underactive thyroid.

Ferritin is stored iron that encourages hairs to grow to their full length. When you aren't getting enough of this mineral through your diet, the body takes ferritin stored in the hair bulb and gives it to essential tissue such as your heart. This leaching of ferritin can cause your hair to shed before it reaches its maximum length eventually leading to hair loss. A 2013 study showed that men with MPB had considerably lower levels of serum ferritin compared to controls, although these were still within the normal range.[29]

Vitamin C helps with absorption while both coffee and tea inhibit uptake. Plant-based sources are less available to the body than iron from foods of animal origin. Grass-fed red meat and liver, green leafy vegetables, lentils, sea vegetables and parsley are all good sources.

Having enough iron is important though more is not necessarily better. High levels are detrimental and tend to accumulate in the tissues of men throughout a lifetime. This ferritin continually damages cells by oxidative stress possibly leading to lipid peroxidation.[30] It also promotes inflammation in the colon, damages the liver and depletes vitamin E. If you have high levels then you can stop eating all processed foods 'fortified' with this mineral; stop taking any vitamins and mineral supplements that contain iron; reduce your intake of animal protein especially red meat; and increase your intake of vitamin E which may be a useful antidote for iron toxicity.[31]

Selenium

This mineral is essential for your thyroid and without selenium there would be no activation of thyroid hormone. In one study 468 infertile men were investigated and researchers found that supplementing with selenium caused an increase in testosterone, among other benefits.[32] This mineral also inhibits mercury and fluoride accumulation, as well as helping the excretion of both mercury and arsenic from the body.[33]

A deficiency in selenium is relatively common. Modern farming practices deplete this mineral from the soil and so is often lacking in our diets. Generally, a little is all that is needed when you consider one Brazil nut is said to be an adequate daily dose. Macadamia nuts, garlic, grass-fed butter, wild mushrooms, mustard seed, ginger, parsley and sea vegetables are other good sources. Make sure you are getting enough zinc in your diet as well, as a deficiency can lead to selenium being used in its place. Amalgam dental fillings may also contribute to a deficiency.[34] Do not take this mineral as a supplement as high levels can also lead to hair loss.[9]

Vitamin D

"Let's not forget that sunlight plain old makes you feel better—not something to be dismissed in the high-stress world in which many of us live. Those who heed warnings to avoid the sun because 'sunlight is dangerous' are robbed of the life-sustaining benefits of sun exposure—and the idea that sunlight is dangerous denies basic evolutionary science…a regular, moderate amount of unprotected sun exposure is absolutely necessary for good health." Michael F. Holick, The Vitamin D Solution

Vitamin D is actually a hormone and, contrary to popular belief, it isn't just about strong bones and teeth. The relationship between vitamin D and testosterone was analysed in 2,299 men.[35] Men with high levels of vitamin D generally had elevated levels of testosterone and vice versa. This research also reported a seasonal pattern, with both vitamin D and testosterone being at their lowest at the end of the winter and peaking at the end of the summer. There is a direct correlation between an elevation in testosterone production and an increase in sun exposure.

This vitamin is important in the prevention of calcification by maintaining the balance of calcium and phosphorus. It also acts as a powerful antioxidant,[36] increases production of another antioxidant superoxide dismutase, promotes regular sleep patterns[37] and reduces the negative effects of stress. Metabolic syndrome is associated with a deficiency.

A 2012 study also indicated that vitamin D helps the dermal papilla cells produce hair follicles.[38] A healthy level is essential for optimal growth and several studies have shown low levels are associated with various types of hair loss.[39,40,41]

Many men are chronically deficient including those with hair loss. In the US it is estimated that around 40 percent of men are deficient. The *2nd National Report on Biochemical Indicators of Diet and Nutrition in the US Population* from 2012 revealed that 8.1 percent of Americans have a *severe* vitamin D deficiency. Between 1988 and 1994, 45 percent of 18,883 people tested in the US had 30 ng/mL or more; a decade later, just 23 percent of 13,369 of those surveyed had at least that amount.[42] The number of men with vitamin D deficiency is on the rise.

This deficiency is caused by the fact that many people work and spend a lot of their leisure time indoors. Air pollution can also be a factor. The best way to optimize your vitamin D levels is from sun exposure. As far as the optimal length of exposure is concerned, you need only enough to have around fifteen to twenty minutes a day with about 40 percent of your skin surface exposed. Some will need less, others more. Sun exposure to the skin is our natural and most effective source. It is impossible to generate too much vitamin D in your body from sunlight exposure: your body will self-regulate and only make what it needs. No research has shown that regular non-burning exposure to UV light poses a significant risk of skin damage though, of course, too much sun is harmful.

Dietary sources include raw milk and wild fish though you can't get enough from foods and multivitamins alone. The modern diet can also have a negative impact on levels. Anything that lowers calcium and magnesium, both vitamin D cofactors, will also reduce levels. Soda, PUFAs, processed foods, vitamin A supplements and fluoridated water are some of the more obvious culprits.

Vitamin E

This vitamin is also commonly deficient. Vitamin E is actually a group of eight compounds and has been shown to increase both total and free testosterone,[43] as well as to lower prolactin.[44] Men with hair loss generally have lower levels of antioxidants, such as vitamin E, in their scalp area.

A study in 2010 investigated the effect of tocotrienol (vitamin E) supplementation on hair growth (almost exclusively men) suffering from hair loss.[45] Thirty-five adults aged eighteen to fifty-nine, completed the eight-month study. Subjects who took vitamin E supplements showed a greater increase in the number of new hairs grown compared to the placebo group. The researchers concluded that: *"A possible explanation for the effects could be due to the potent antioxidant activity of tocotrienols that help to reduce lipid peroxidation and oxidative stress in the scalp, which are known to be associated with alopecia* [MPB]*."*

Some good dietary sources include olive oil and olives, almonds, avocados, green leafy vegetables and chili pepper. Topical application of castor or coconut oil to the scalp may also be beneficial. Do not take vitamin E as a supplement as this can in the long-term lead to hair loss.[9]

Vitamin A

Not a single vitamin but describes a group of five similar compounds including retinol and beta-carotene (pro-vitamin A). Retinol is generally found in animal foods while beta-carotene is in fruit and vegetables and converted into retinol within the body. Vitamin A is critically important in the development and maintenance of both the hair follicle and sebaceous glands. Either too little or too much of this vitamin can lead to hair loss.

In a 2000 study beta-carotene levels were found to be significantly lower in patients with hair loss.[46] The researchers concluded: *"these results provide some evidence for a potential role of increased lipid peroxidation and decreased antioxidants in alopecia."*

Vitamin A is also needed for the enzymes involved in the synthesis of steroid hormones such as testosterone and so a deficiency will negatively impact their production. Vitamin A also decreases oestrogen production.[47]

There are two kinds of deficiency. In primary deficiency, the individual does not ingest the recommended daily amount either from plant or animal sources. This vitamin breaks down easily when it's cooked or stored for a long time. Secondary deficiency occurs when certain factors affect the optimal absorption from the intestine. These include: zinc or iron deficiency, low stomach acid, food allergies, smoking and excess alcohol. A balance between vitamin A and D is also essential. An excess of one can create a relative deficiency of the other.

Good dietary sources include: grass-fed beef liver, grass-fed butter, green leafy vegetables especially dandelion greens, carrots, sweet potatoes, goji berries and butternut squash. If you eat vitamin A-rich foods along with some fat then the amount absorbed is greatly increased. Do not take vitamin A (or beta-carotene) as a supplement as this can lead to hair loss and a vitamin D deficiency.[9]

Vitamin C (ascorbic acid)

This vitamin has been shown to reduce oxidative stress and cortisol levels, as well as helping to strengthen and thicken hair. An *in vitro* study in 2009 found that a derivative of vitamin C promoted growth of the human hair follicle.[48] Another study tested ninety-two randomly selected healthy adults.[49] They found lipid peroxidation was significantly increased in groups of subjects with deficient levels of vitamin C and/or vitamin E, compared to those with normal levels. The researchers concluded that deficiency in either vitamin C or E resulted in insufficient defence against free radicals and increased lipid peroxidation.

The adrenals need more vitamin C than any other organ or tissue in the body, especially during times of stress. If you are suffering from chronic stress then you likely have low levels. This vitamin improves the absorption of iron and vitamin B_{12}, as well as reducing the affects of phytic acid and mycotoxins. Good dietary sources include green leafy vegetables, citrus fruit, broccoli, berries, guava and papaya. However, this vitamin is easily destroyed during food preparation especially when cooked.

Vitamin K_2

This relatively unknown vitamin has demonstrated a pivotal role in inhibiting calcification[50] as well as lowering levels of oestrogen in the body.[51] A poor diet is one of the main factors that cause a deficiency: but also the use of antibiotics and intestinal problems can decrease the ability to absorb or produce this vitamin. We can partly convert the vitamin K_1 to K_2 by friendly bacteria in the digestive system but this conversion is inefficient: so we benefit much more from eating vitamin K_2 directly. This important nutrient is incredibly low in the modern diet and can be found in grass-fed organ meat, grass-fed butter, natto (fermented soybeans) and fermented vegetables especially red cabbage.

Antioxidants

Oxidative stress and lipid peroxidation can be reduced by antioxidants. Vitamins C, D and E are powerful antioxidants as well as the minerals zinc, magnesium and selenium. Another two important ones relevant to hair loss are superoxide dismutase (SOD) and glutathione.

Superoxide dismutase: As you age the body starts making less of this antioxidant enzyme. However, you can encourage its production by increasing your intake of zinc, manganese, iron and vitamin D. Certain foods have also been shown to elevate levels including: apples, cardamom, cloves, nettle, aloe vera, broccoli sprouts, cruciferous vegetables, sprouted grains and the herbs He shou wu and mucuna pruriens. On the other hand: smoking, high blood sugar, mycotoxins in food[52] and exposure to fluoride[53] can all lead to a reduction in levels.

In a 2016 study patients with MPB had significantly decreased SOD and total antioxidant activity compared to age-matched controls.[54] The researchers concluded these results were indicators of oxidative stress.

In a 2012 study the researchers had this to say: *"Because this enzyme is a very potent antioxidant, SOD combats the effects of free radicals that are causing hair follicles to die."*[55]

Glutathione: This antioxidant is usually produced in the body, though there are some dietary sources including spinach, asparagus, avocado and fermented foods. Apart from protecting hair follicles from oxidative damage and lipid peroxidation, glutathione is involved in the detoxification of substances such as mercury. It is also an essential cofactor in the conversion of active thyroid hormone. Environmental pollutants such as toxic heavy metals, poor diet, an unhealthy gut microbiome, pharmaceutical drugs like acetaminophen/paracetamol and excessive stress all reduce levels.

In a 2000 study glutathione was found to be significantly lower in patients with hair loss than in controls.[46] They also found levels of oxidative stress were higher. These results indicated that antioxidants such as glutathione play a critical role in preventing MPB.

Glutathione is comprised largely of three amino acids: cysteine, glutamine and glycine. Supplies of cysteine are the rate-limiting factor in glutathione synthesis, since it is relatively rare in food. Sulphur-rich vegetables such as garlic, leeks and onions/shallots as well as cruciferous vegetables are all rich sources in addition to red bell peppers, artichoke and parsley. The herbs rosemary, turmeric, He shou wu, mucuna pruriens and milk thistle can stimulate production as well as foods containing the phytonutrient resveratrol. Magnesium is essential for glutathione production while both vitamin C and selenium are needed for its activity within the body.

Phytonutrients

Plant foods contain natural chemical compounds called phytonutrients (phytochemicals) that are not considered nutrients essential for life. They protect plants from insects, disease, inclement weather and browsing animals. When we eat them, the very same protective compounds are made available to our bodies. More than eight thousand different phytonutrients have been identified to date and each plant produces several hundred.

Whilst there is no formal recommendation for phytonutrients, the best way to obtain them is from a varied diet. Unfortunately, not only has the quality of food we eat lessened but also the variety. I recommend consuming a wide range of fruits, vegetables, herbs and spices to get all the phytonutrients you need as well as eating organic and wild foods. With regard to hair growth, a few phytonutrients may be of particular importance:

Quercetin: In a 2012 study researchers found that quercetin injections prevented or reduced spontaneous onset of hair loss in mice.[56] This phytonutrient has also been reported to possess strong anti-inflammatory capacities, specifically reducing the effects of TNF.[57] Several phytonutrients have been demonstrated to be natural aromatase inhibitors including quercetin, apigenin and naringenin.[58]

Heating, especially boiling, significantly reduces the amount of this phytonutrient so aim to eat quercetin-rich foods that are either raw or only lightly cooked. Good sources include: green and black tea, capers, lovage, radish leaves, rocket (arugula), onions/shallots and parsley.

Kaempferol: In a 2017 study this phytonutrient was found to promote hair growth and increased the proliferation of dermal papilla cells significantly more than the hair loss drug minoxidil.[59] Kaempferol has also been shown to possess anti-inflammatory activity including reduction of prostaglandins and TNF.[60]

This phytonutrient is found in many foods and herbs including: aloe vera, rosemary, basil, great burnet, horsetail, coriander, apples, green tea, onions/shallots and leeks.

Myricetin: This phytonutrient has anti-inflammatory[61] and antioxidant properties exceeding that of vitamin E.[62] Myricetin has also been shown to decrease blood glucose and triglyceride levels.[63]

Good sources of myricetin include parsley, guava, grapes, onions/shallots, broccoli, berries, rutabaga (swede) and spinach.

Naringenin: This phytonutrient is an aromatase inhibitor as well as a reducer of oxidative stress in the hair follicle. In a 2017 study researchers investigated the *in vitro* effects on human dermal papilla and skin cells.[64] They found naringenin significantly increased the proliferation of both types of cell, suggesting protection against oxidative stress associated with hair loss. This phytonutrient has also been shown to prevent liver inflammation, necrosis (premature cell death) and fibrosis, owing to its antioxidant capacity.[65]

Good sources of this phytonutrient include citrus fruits such as bitter orange, tangerine, lime, bergamot and lemon as well as tart cherries, cacao and tomatoes.

Apigenin: A 2009 *in vitro* study discovered that apigenin stimulated the elongation of hair follicles.[66] The findings suggested that this phytonutrient, which is known to have antioxidant and anti-inflammatory properties, stimulates hair growth by repressing TGF-beta1. In another study, several phytonutrients were screened for their aromatase inhibiting properties. The greatest activity was demonstrated with apigenin.[67]

Good sources of this phytonutrient include parsley, celery, rosemary, thyme, oregano, basil, chamomile and cloves.

Luteolin: This phytonutrient has been shown to reduce greatly both acute and chronic inflammation.[68] Luteolin may also block the aromatase enzyme or inhibit its synthesis. It has been shown to be a potent aromatase inhibitor without the side effects of a drug commonly used to lower this enzyme.[69]

Good sources of luteolin include dried oregano, celery seed, thyme, radicchio, celery, broccoli, parsley, dandelion leaves, chamomile and rosemary.

Resveratrol: The powerful anti-inflammatory properties of this phytonutrient include inhibiting the synthesis of both PGD_2[70] and TNF.[71] Resveratrol is also a potent antioxidant, helps induce the synthesis of glutathione and is an effective aromatase inhibitor.[72]

Good sources of resveratrol include Japanese knotweed, red grapes, cacao and berries such as blueberries and mulberries.

Salicin (salicylic acid): This phytonutrient was originally extracted from the bark of the white willow tree and later synthetically produced to become the common drug aspirin. It is an inhibitor of oxidative stress, reduces high blood sugar and derivatives have been found to be potent anti-oestrogen agents.[73] Researchers have stated that: *"The most famous and defined effect of salicylic acid is prostaglandin synthesis inhibition. Salicylic acid has anti-inflammatory effects…is a confirmed inhibitor of oxidative stress…we can conclude that salicylic acid is a potent and important naturally occurring phytochemical with numerous health-promoting effects."*[74]

Apart from white willow bark this phytonutrient is also found in the herbs meadowsweet, sweet and white birch, wintergreen and poplar. Herbs are the preferred choice as they have fewer side effects than drugs and are more readily excreted from the body. So, try to get this phytonutrient from natural sources rather than a pill.

Procyanidin B2: In a 2002 animal study scientists found procyanidin B2 promoted hair growth.[75] This phytonutrient was shown to activate the growth cycle of hair follicles while decreasing the resting phase. Procyanidin B2 has also been shown to suppress oestrogen synthesis both *in vitro* and *in vivo*.[76]

Good dietary sources include cinnamon, hawthorn flowers, cat's claw, grape leaves, lychee (litchi) and apples (especially crab apples).

Procyanidin B3: A 2002 study demonstrated that this phytonutrient can directly promote hair cell growth and stimulate the growth phase of follicles by inhibiting TGF-beta1.[77] Procyanidin B3 has also been shown to possess strong anti-inflammatory activity.[78]

Good dietary sources of this phytonutrient include pine bark, red grapes, barley, peaches and the young branch stems of the South American plant huanarpo macho.

The beneficial effects of phytonutrients with regard to hair growth include: reducing aromatase activity, increasing growth of dermal papilla cells, improving blood glucose levels as well as powerful antioxidant and anti-inflammatory effects. Many everyday herbs and spices are excellent sources such as oregano, rosemary, thyme, basil and parsley. A meta-analysis showed that phytonutrients were significantly higher in organic crops than conventional.[79] Just like vitamins, I do not recommend taking concentrated doses far higher than you find anywhere in nature. Given that there are hundreds of phytonutrients in each plant, it is extremely difficult to isolate any one single ingredient that is solely responsible for one particular effect. Rather than get overexcited from a single study of one compound, I think it is better to focus on eating a wide range of foods and herbs.

Getting Tested for Nutrients

If you are suffering from a nutritional deficiency then this shortage should be corrected. The only way to know for certain is to get tested. Checking that your vitamin and mineral levels are optimum is a sensible precautionary measure, although it is not possible to test for all essential nutrients or phytonutrients. Laboratory reference ranges differ but generally aim for the high end. The following blood tests are all recommended:

Minerals and trace elements: zinc, copper and iron (ferritin). The ideal range of serum ferritin lies between 40-60 ng/mL. If your ferritin is too high, speak to your doctor about the possibility of donating blood to help reduce your level. You can also test for selenium, but this is usually quite expensive.

Vitamins: A, B_1, B_2, B_3, B_5, B_6, B_7 (biotin), B_9 (folate), B_{12}, C and E.

Antioxidants: CoQ_{10} and glutathione.

Iodine: For an iodine deficiency it is best to check your thyroid.

Magnesium: A blood serum test for magnesium is not accurate, so you can order a sublingual epithelial test.

Vitamin D: Correct blood test for vitamin D status is 25-hydroxycholecaliferol or 25-hydroxyvitamin D (25 OH vitamin D). A level of around 48 ng/mL is preferable. 1,25-dihydroxyvitamin D is NOT the correct test.

PTH and calcium: PTH measures the level of parathyroid hormone in the blood. PTH should always be requested with calcium as it is not just the amounts of each that are important. The balance between them is significant and the response of the parathyroid glands to changing concentration of calcium. High blood (serum) calcium concentrations may be owing to overproduction of PTH by the parathyroid glands.

Body Systems

Multiple organs perform together to keep your body operating. These body systems are all interconnected and dependent upon one another to function. Even seemingly unrelated systems are connected and work together to maintain internal stability and balance: problems in one can cause trouble in another. As well as the thyroid, your adrenals, liver and digestive system are all responsible for the health of your hair.

Adrenals

You have a pair of triangular-shaped glands sitting on top of your kidneys called the adrenals. These help your body to manage and survive during stressful situations. They also produce nearly 50 percent of all the androgens in your body, including around 5 percent of testosterone. Under continued stress, the adrenals become overactive and will release high, constant levels of stress hormones such as cortisol. Your adrenals respond to every kind of stress in the same way whatever the source, whether it is chemical, physical or emotional. The effects are cumulative, even when the individual stressors are quite different or whether or not you recognise them as stressors.

Apart from cortisol other adrenal hormones have been implicated in hair loss. DHEA and its sulphated form DHEA-S both act as a hormone precursor for oestrogen and testosterone. In a 2020 study forty-three men with early onset MPB were found to have increased levels of DHEA-S and at least one of the following: high body mass index, insulin resistance or low SHBG.[80] The researchers concluded that: elevated insulin levels led to an increase in DHEA-S, a decrease in total testosterone and a reduction in blood supply to hair follicles.

In an earlier 1987 study eighteen men aged between eighteen and thirty-two with rapidly progressive hair loss had their levels of testosterone and DHEA-S measured.[81] The men with MPB had significantly higher levels of DHEA-S compared to controls. The researchers suggested adrenal hyperactivity initiated hair loss.

A 1991 study looked at sixty-five patients with hair loss and also concluded that overactive adrenal glands were involved in MPB.[82]

These studies are all indicating that higher levels of stress hormones are associated with MPB. One of the most common causes of high DHEA or DHEA-S is constant and persistent daily stress. As part of your overall plan to prevent hair loss it is essential to start reducing chronic stress and decrease adrenal activity.

Another adrenal hormone, aldosterone, has been implicated in the development of MPB. Aldosterone helps regulate your blood pressure by managing the balance of potassium and sodium in the body. In a 2013 study thirty men with MPB showed significantly higher aldosterone and blood pressure values compared to controls.[83] The researchers concluded that: "*Aldosterone might have a role in the pathogenesis of AGA* [development of MPB] *and its serum level is related to disease severity.*" This may help to explain the association between MPB and elevated blood pressure.

A deficiency in magnesium, calcium, vitamin D or potassium produces higher levels of this hormone. This leads to an increase in parathyroid hormone and prolactin, which in turn can initiate calcification. Aldosterone also causes an elevation in ROS and TGF-beta1, leading to increased oxidative stress and inflammation.

Usually problems with these glands are caused by chronic stress, blood sugar imbalances or gut inflammation. The health of the adrenals affects thyroid function and vice versa, so you also need to make sure your thyroid is working well. You can nurture your kidneys and adrenals by drinking plenty of filtered or spring water and eating foods such as olives, avocados, coconut oil and green leafy vegetables. The herbs ashwagandha, hydrangea root, tulsi (holy basil) and valerian root may also be beneficial. It's best to avoid excess caffeine and other stimulants especially when you are fatigued and stressed, along with processed and fried foods.

Liver

This organ plays an enormous role in the detoxification process. The fewer toxins you are exposed to, the less work your liver has to do. Conversely, our bodies are not always functioning at an optimal level and are unable to properly dispose of all the harmful chemicals we encounter. The liver can be overloaded by overeating, illness, poor nutrition, stress, pollution as well as recreational and medicinal drugs. Pharmaceuticals are not evolutionarily natural to the human body. Prescription drugs should be a last resort if any kind of health issue arises. Find out if there are natural remedies that your doctor recommends to replace current medications you may be taking.

The liver controls the production of hormones such as active thyroid hormone and the breakdown of others like cortisol and oestrogen. The liver requires the B-complex vitamins (especially B_6 and B_{12}) and magnesium to break down and deactivate oestrogen. High cortisol levels or a disruption of the supply of glucose will prevent this organ's ability to clear excess oestrogen from the blood.

It is important to support detoxification pathways with certain foods and herbs as well as regular exercise. Your liver requires high levels of sulphur, and this is found in foods such as: green beans, radish, parsley, watercress, cabbage, onion/shallots and garlic. Other good foods for the liver include: ginger, beets, carrots, citrus fruits and Jerusalem artichokes. Herbs such as thyme, oregano, rosemary, milk thistle, turmeric and dandelion root are all beneficial in supporting the liver as well as gallbladder and bile duct function.

Digestive System
"All disease begins in the gut." Hippocrates

We consume somewhere around thirty to sixty tons of food in our lifetime. The digestive system must function in an optimal fashion to be able to process and absorb all of this food as well as keeping toxins from entering the body. The flora of the gut, composed of approximately one hundred billion bacteria, is collectively known as the microbiome: and the importance of a healthy microbiome cannot be overstated. If it is unbalanced, it becomes one of the main culprits behind inflammation throughout the whole body. It is possible that reducing inflammation in the gut could reduce the expression of inflammation in the hair follicles. I believe that making sure your digestive system and microbiome are functioning well is essential for the health of your hair.

The composition of the microbiome can be altered by diet.[84] Unfortunately, unbalanced gut bacteria is common today owing to: diets high in conventionally raised meat and dairy products, processed foods, antibiotics, antacids, exposure to toxic chemicals as well as chronic stress.[85] An unhealthy microbiome has been shown to cause both insulin resistance and inflammation.[86] Researchers found that almost a quarter of people they studied had 40 percent fewer bacteria than would normally be expected in a healthy gut.[87] The ones they did have were more likely to cause inflammation than the health-promoting bacteria. It has recently been hypothesized that stress exposure may directly upset the microbiome. During periods of stress more inflammation-producing bacteria begin to thrive and good bacteria start to disappear.[88]

Disruption of healthy bacteria results in the reduction of beneficial byproducts such as vitamin B_{12} as well as the increased production of disease-causing bacteria and their waste products (endotoxins). These endotoxins exert a tremendous inflammatory response in the body by stimulating the release of prostaglandins[89] and cause the liver to produce more TNF. In addition they increase oestrogen by activating the aromatase enzyme,[90] lower glutathione levels,[91] negatively affect thyroid function[92] and elevate cortisol. Normally, our intestine and liver destroy most of these endotoxins before they reach the general circulation. But if the health of your digestive tract and liver are compromised then more endotoxins will be absorbed. The best way to reduce exposure is to keep your microbiome balanced.

In one study scientists discovered that a rapid decline in testosterone production occurred in healthy men following administration of low-dose endotoxin.[93] Exposure reduced testosterone production by 30 percent within just six hours. This confirmed the interaction between endotoxin exposure, subsequent inflammation and impaired testicular function in men. An unhealthy microbiome may therefore be partly responsible for lowering testosterone levels.

The liver has long been recognised as the primary organ of detoxification but there is now growing evidence that the gut also plays a central role in this process. Oestrogen is metabolized by the liver and cleared out of the body through the bowel. If it encounters the wrong type of bacteria in the bowel, this hormone can be readily reabsorbed and not excreted. An important factor in decreasing your level of oestrogen is therefore improvement in gut health.

You can enhance digestive health and lessen the effects of endotoxins by reducing your intake of conventionally produced meat or dairy. These contain inevitable traces of antibiotics that indiscriminately kill the beneficial bacteria in your digestive system. Any preservatives added to packaged and processed food such as sulfites essentially do the same thing. These chemicals are meant to make a food edible for many years by eliminating any bacteria and other microbes. When they enter your body, they will do the same in your gut. Avoid drinking chlorinated tap water as this can also destroy friendly bacteria. For the same reasons, do not take antibiotics unless absolutely essential as these substances eliminate microbes all over the body including your digestive system. If you cannot avoid their use, take care to consume probiotics both during the course and for several weeks afterward.

Several studies have shown that heavy meat eaters, as compared to vegans, vegetarians and occasional meat eaters have a less healthy microbiome, though categorizing people based on these choices alone is somewhat oversimplified. Researchers studying the faecal microbiome of omnivores, vegetarians and vegans concluded: *"Overall, these findings confirm that, type of food consumed more that the dietary habits or geographical origin, can have an impact on fecal microbio*[me]*."*[94] In other words, the quality of what you eat is important for a healthy microbiome rather than a single ideal diet.

Probiotics and prebiotics are fantastic for your digestive system and help to reduce endotoxins. Probiotics are beneficial live bacteria that are either the same or very similar to those already in your body. Good choices of probiotics include raw sauerkraut, raw apple cider vinegar and raw grass-fed dairy. Prebiotics, like inulin, are specialized plant fibres that feed the good bacteria already in the gut and help raise their number. While probiotics introduce bacteria into the gut, prebiotics act as a fertilizer for those already there. Some foods that are high in prebiotics include chicory root, Jerusalem artichokes, leeks, onions/shallots, dandelion root, burdock root, carrot and jicama. Herbs such as cat's claw, wormwood, marshmallow, cloves and thyme are also beneficial for your digestive system.

A lack of sufficient stomach acid results in poor digestion of many nutrients. Too much acid is a very rare condition while too little acid is common. Proper stomach acid production is critical to the rest of the digestive process, so it's an issue to address. The vast majority of people who suffer reflux and heartburn actually don't produce enough acid in their stomach and antacids make the problem worse. Jonathon Wright, author and doctor, estimates that approximately 90 percent of Americans produce too little stomach acid. *"In twenty-four years of nutritionally oriented practice, I've worked with thousands of individuals who've found the cause of their heartburn and indigestion to be low stomach acidity."*

Several factors are responsible for low stomach acid including: chronic stress and anxiety; food allergy, intolerance or sensitivity;

nutritional deficiencies including zinc and vitamins B_1 and C; overeating; inappropriate food combination; excess alcohol consumption; diets high in processed food. Apart from addressing these issues you can also increase your consumption of bitter foods, fermented foods and natural acids such as citrus fruits. Other factors that may be helpful in improving your digestion include: not rushing through meals; not working while eating; chewing food slowly; not drinking cold fluids with food and drinking a tablespoon of raw apple cider vinegar before any meal. There are two books that I recommend to help you gain an understanding of food combining: Kimberly Snyder's *The Beauty Detox Solution* and Daniel Reid's *The Tao of Health, Sex and Longevity*. Another book I recommend to understand issues with your digestive system is Dr Michael Ruscio's *Healthy Gut, Healthy You*.

Getting Your Body Systems Tested

Adrenals: Refer to stress and inflammation. Iron deficiency often goes along with an inadequate adrenal response as well as an underactive thyroid. An electrolyte panel measures the blood levels of sodium, potassium, chloride and carbon dioxide and helps in diagnosing any adrenal problems.

Liver: Liver function tests check for liver damage and can help diagnose any liver or bile duct problems.

Digestive System: A gastrointestinal profile test (gastrointestinal pathogens panel) will access your gut health including levels of bacteria, yeast, fungus and parasites. It also reveals important information about the production of digestive enzymes.

You may not even realise you have sensitivities to some of the foods you eat on a regular basis. A food allergy blood panel can show exactly which ones may be an issue. Salivary tests (www.cyrexlabs.com), a stool antigen test (www.enterolab.com) or analysis of your microbiome (www.viome.com) can reveal any problems with reasonable accuracy.

Your stomach acid can be checked directly though this is usually expensive. Alternatively check chloride levels. Low blood levels (under 100 mEq/L) are a sign of low stomach acid.

Part 4: Food and Herbs

"Don't make yourself miserable in your attempt to be healthy."
Dr Michael Ruscio, Healthy Gut, Healthy You

Many men are interested in eating more healthily but making such a change can sometimes be difficult. Some men also fear appearing different from other people with regard to diet. They think changing their food choices will result in a loss or weakening of their social relationships possibly with regard to their 'manliness.' Real men would not be caught dead eating a large salad. The first step in eliminating any habit is to make a firm decision to break it. Incorporating new healthier choices one at a time is the way. Trying to rush and do too many things at once will just result in becoming overwhelmed. Make gradual changes and you'll eventually drop your bad dietary ways.

A nutritious diet is the backbone of any regime for healthy hair and it's important to eat well to reduce inflammation and balance blood sugar. Not only should you improve your regular diet by consuming more fresh fruit and vegetables and less processed food but also try less obvious choices such as fermented foods and seaweeds as well as eating organic and wild foods.

Vegetables and Herbs

Leafy Green Vegetables: Raw leafy greens are both high in antioxidants and also help to reduce inflammation. Good choices include kale, spring greens, spinach, Swiss chard, rocket and beet greens (leafy greens attached to beet roots). Always choose organic spring greens (collards) and kale, not because they contain a large number of pesticides but because, according to the *Environmental Working Group's* report from 2017, they are sprayed with the most toxic ones. Spinach has potentially high pesticide contamination so, again, try to buy organic.

Spinach, beet greens and Swiss chard all contain the anti-nutrient oxalate (oxalic acid). Oxalate can bind to calcium in the gut and prevent some of it from being absorbed. It is true that this anti-nutrient in the diet reduces one's effective intake of calcium but the size of the effect is relatively small and not meaningful. This is not a reason to avoid them. If desired, you may cook these greens to reduce some of their oxalate content.

Some less common varieties of green leafy vegetables that you can incorporate into your diet include:

Watercress: Part of the cruciferous family, watercress contains more vitamin C than oranges, more calcium than whole milk and more iron than spinach. This green is fantastic in a salad or a juice to give a peppery bite. Scientists ranked forty-one vegetables and fruits for nutrient potential and watercress came out on top.[1] Others highly ranked were bok choy, Swiss chard, beet greens and spinach.

Nettle: When you consider eating your greens, this is probably not what you first think of. This amazing plant is usually referred to as stinging nettle, though this activity is lost when the plant is dried, cooked or juiced. Nettle exhibits strong antioxidant activity,[2] reduces aromatase, inhibits prostaglandins and contains high levels of silica and more protein than any other land plant.

You can steam them just like spinach or add to a smoothie or juice. The leaves, either fresh or dried, can also be used to make tea. Pick your own wild nettle: the tender tops of young plants are delicious and nutritious. The best way not to get stung is to wear gloves or simply snip them into a container with scissors. Collect the leaves before they flower in spring.

Dandelion greens: Everything, from the flower all the way down to the roots, is edible. This 'weed' is actually incredibly nutritious and a good source of magnesium, calcium, beta-carotene, vitamin C and the phytonutrient luteolin. Dandelion promotes liver function and supports the growth of beneficial bacteria in the digestive system. According to a *New York Times* article, wild dandelions have about seven times more phytonutrients than store-bought spinach.[3]

Broccoli: This cruciferous vegetable is an exceptionally rich source of vitamin C and other antioxidants. Broccoli supports the digestive system, prevents oxidative stress and reduces inflammation. Both the leaves and stalk can be added to a juice. A derivative of a chemical found in cruciferous vegetables (such as broccoli, cauliflower and cabbage) has been shown to interfere with aromatase activity.[4] Sulforaphane, another compound found in cruciferous vegetables and their sprouts, has been demonstrated to inhibit the production of TNF.[5]

Asparagus: This distinct and delicious vegetable is best eaten fresh as it loses nutrients and flavour rapidly. It promotes the growth of beneficial bacteria in the gut and is a good source of beta-carotene, vitamins C and B_9 (folate) and chromium. Asparagus is also particularly high in the phytonutrients quercetin and kaempferol as well as containing the antioxidant glutathione.

Parsnips: This root vegetable is a great source of soluble fibre as well as androstenol and boron, which both help to increase levels of testosterone. They are often overlooked when it comes to making a vegetable juice but have a sweet taste similar to carrot but with its own distinctive flavour. Parsnips can also be fermented.

Radish: Bulbs come in many shapes and colours such as red radish, daikon, black radish and horseradish. They are anti-inflammatory, antimicrobial, stimulate secretion of digestive enzymes and increase the flow of bile, so helping to maintain a healthy liver. Radishes can also diminish or prevent the effects of mycotoxins in the digestive system.[6] Try to buy with their greens still attached. These are an excellent source of the phytonutrient quercetin and can be eaten in a salad or juiced. Radishes are also great to ferment.

Chili peppers: Some of the most popular varieties include bell peppers, cayenne and jalapeno. Whether eaten fresh, dried or powdered (paprika) they are excellent sources of vitamin C as well as capsaicin which possesses antioxidant, anti-bacterial and anti-diabetic properties. Always choose organic chili peppers: according to the 2018 *Environmental Working Group's* report, they are sprayed with the most toxic pesticides.

Celery: This vegetable is high in fibre and antioxidants that are known to be anti-inflammatory including the phytonutrient luteolin (a powerful aromatase inhibitor). Conventional celery has also been shown to contain significant amounts of pesticide traces so always try to buy organic. The leaves as well as the stalks can be juiced.

Onions/Shallots: These pungent vegetables are rich in sulphur-containing compounds, which are the primary source of their strong smell. Onions have been shown to increase significantly total testosterone[7] as well as possibly lowering blood sugar levels.[8] You get the most benefits when they are consumed raw and the smaller the onion is, the stronger its flavour will be. Ounce-for-ounce shallots have around six times more phytonutrients than the typical onion.

Leeks: A member of the onion family but with a sweeter, more subtle flavour. Like onions they provide a good source of inulin, a soluble fibre that feeds the good bacteria in your digestive system. Leeks also have anti-bacterial, anti-viral and anti-fungal properties.

Beetroot: Try buying with the greens attached as these can be eaten as well. Beetroot displays potent antioxidant and anti-inflammatory activity.[9]

Sweet Potatoes: These starchy root vegetables are an excellent source of beta-carotene, vitamin C and manganese. Sweet potatoes have also been shown to promote the growth of beneficial bacteria in the gut.

Aloe Vera: This desert plant's use can be traced back thousands of years to early Egypt where it was known as the 'plant of immortality.' Aloe gel is the clear, jelly-like substance found in the inner part of the leaf. To use, cut a three to four-inch section, trim off the spikes, slice in half and scoop out the clear gel with a spoon. This is great in either a smoothie or juice. Aloe vera is antimicrobial and anti-inflammatory[10] when used both externally as well as internally. In addition, this plant has been shown to: decrease blood glucose and improve lipid profiles in pre-diabetic patients,[11] inhibit prostaglandin production[12] and increase levels of the antioxidant SOD.[13] Try to find fresh aloe vera and make this incredible plant part of your diet.

Garlic: This plant is antimicrobial without harming beneficial gut bacteria, promotes healthy digestion, reduces the stress hormone cortisol and stimulates blood circulation to your scalp. Garlic has also been shown to increase production of testosterone whilst lowering cortisol levels in rats fed a high protein diet.[14]

Ginger: This root has many positive health benefits and to make the most of its virtues you should use fresh root, not powder. Ginger increases total testosterone levels[15] and reduces inflammation as well as the production of pro-inflammatory chemicals known to cause hair loss.[16,17] It has also been demonstrated to reduce lipid peroxidation and oxidative stress by modulating the levels of antioxidants including glutathione.[18]

Turmeric: This bright yellow root has: antibacterial and antifungal properties; acts as a digestive stimulant; helps to reduce stress; lowers both oxidative stress and lipid peroxidation[19] and suppresses increases in blood sugar levels.[20] The active ingredient has been shown to be a potent inhibitor of the inflammatory cytokine TNF,[21] as well as inhibiting both prostaglandin synthesis[22] and TGF-beta1 signalling.[23] Simply put, turmeric inhibits several chemicals known to cause hair loss.
Eating turmeric with fat and black pepper increases its bioavailability. Turmeric powder often isn't very fresh, possibly contaminated with mould, and sometimes made with harsh processes that destroy or degrade its healthful components. Use fresh root if you can find it.

The following herbs are also all wonderful to add to your regular food and juices: black pepper, parsley, coriander (cilantro), oregano, thyme, basil, rosemary, dill and bay leaves. We usually think of herbs and spices as nothing more than taste enhancers but they are an incredible source of phytonutrients and antioxidants. Throw out any old herbs and spices. Use high quality, fresh herbs and spices or don't use them at all. Many commercial varieties are irradiated so buy organic or, better still, grow a few in your kitchen or garden.

Vegetable Juice

A large glass of fresh juice a day is a great way to add a wider variety of vegetables to your diet. Good choices include cucumber, celery, green leafy vegetables like kale and spinach, bell pepper, parsley, turmeric, ginger, onion, radish and beetroot. The best time is between meals on an empty stomach for optimal absorption. Any leftovers from your cooking such as broccoli stems, radish leaves or parsley stalks can be saved and added to a juice.

Those available in stores such as *V8*, *Tropicana* and other pre-packaged, pre-bottled drinks are not recommended. They can be stored in holding tanks for up to a year before being packaged. The nature of the bottling process means that most have been pasteurized. This involves heating to such high temperatures that the enzymes and much of the nutrition have been destroyed. The juices can also be stored in cartons that leach phthalates (a known hormone disruptor).

Fruit
"In my estimation, fruit is the ideal carbohydrate source." Danny Roddy, *Hair Like a Fox*

The desire for sweet-tasting foods is perfectly normal and natural. Indeed, our tongue contains an abundance of sweet receptors for a good reason. Fresh ripe fruit supplies you with readily available energy that can be used for immediate fuel, as well as water, vitamins, minerals, fibre and phytonutrients. Many people now believe that because added sugars are bad, the same must apply to fruit, which contains fructose. The human body is well adapted to the small amounts found in whole fruit which doesn't provoke an insulin response. Then again, concentrated fructose in high-fructose corn syrup and other artificial sweeteners can cause a real health problem and should be avoided.

Low doses of fructose have been shown to improve glucose tolerance in adults with type 2 diabetes as well as normal adults.[24] So long as you are eating a healthy diet then fruit will not cause any issues with glucose metabolism or insulin sensitivity. It can however be a problem in people if their diet is rich in PUFA, refined carbohydrate and processed food. Fruit and fructose just magnify the problems of a bad diet.

The definition of a fruit is that it bears its own seed. 'Seedless' varieties have been genetically tampered with and are higher in sugar while lower in minerals. Instead go for natural varieties, which bear their own seeds, just as nature intended.

Citrus: The nutritional benefits of limes do not differ very much from those of lemons. Both are strongly antibacterial and antimicrobial as well as having significant antioxidant and anti-inflammatory effects, including the inhibition of TNF.[25] Ounce-for-ounce, the peels have many times more phytonutrients than the flesh. Most of the pesticide residues are in the skin, so consume only if you buy organic.

Avocado: This highly versatile fruit is perfect to add to a salad and has a moderating effect on bitter tastes such as leafy greens. This fruit can also be added to a smoothie giving a fluffy and creamy consistency. Avocados are one of the few foods that contain significant levels of vitamin C and E, as well as the antioxidant glutathione. They are the richest known fruit source of plant sterols, which may indirectly help to lower oestrogen levels. This fruit has also been demonstrated to reduce both oxidative stress and inflammation.[26]

Berries: Good choices include blueberries, blackberries, mulberries, cranberries, raspberries and goji berries. Blueberries have been shown to improve insulin sensitivity[27] and reduce prolactin levels.[28] Goji berries are most commonly available in dried form and contain high amounts of beta-carotene. They have been shown to decrease significantly blood sugar levels.[29]

Pomegranate: This fruit is a potent antioxidant containing quercetin, luteolin and vitamin C. Pomegranate has been shown to: inhibit the enzyme aromatase;[30] increase salivary testosterone levels;[31] improve lipid profiles;[32] reduce blood pressure and lipid peroxidation and decrease the production of the inflammatory chemical TNF.[33]

Olives: A good source of vitamin E and monounsaturated fats. Both green and black olives (as well as olive oil) help to reduce inflammation in the body.[34] Look for those with the pits intact and sold fresh or in a glass jar and not a can or in plastic.

Coconut: The white flesh inside a coconut is a good source of manganese, selenium and zinc. This fruit has been shown to reduce inflammation, improve gut bacteria[35] and lower blood sugar levels.[36]

Apples: This fruit has been shown to increase antioxidant activity in the body including raising levels of SOD.[37] They are also a good source of vitamin C, soluble fibre and the phytonutrient procyanidin B2. Try buying organic as apples are close to the top of the list of produce most contaminated with pesticides. Many of these chemicals are applied after the harvest, so they can have a longer shelf life.

Other great fruit choices include fig, guava, papaya (pawpaw) and prickly pear (cactus fruit).

Sea Vegetables (seaweed)

Although we associate sea vegetables with Asian cuisine, many sea-bordering countries have traditionally included them in their diet and they are amongst the most nutritious foods on the planet. They are an excellent source of iodine, reduce inflammation and blood sugar levels,[38] improve the gut microbiome and possess antioxidant properties.[39]

Sea vegetables are usually found in dried pieces though you can also buy them in powder or tablet form. Try and buy organic as many commercial varieties are treated with pesticides and fungicides. Soak dry pieces for about five minutes in filtered water and then drain and squeeze out the excess liquid before you eat them. Each variety has its own unique flavour. If you try one and don't like it, don't dismiss them all. They are great in soups and mixed with rice.

Kelp: The most readily available type of edible seaweed with kombu and wakame being popular forms. Kelp is extremely high in iodine. Although it looks like a plant, kelp is a protista (assorted group of microorganisms). One teaspoon of powder has approximately one thousand times more calcium than a 250 ml glass of milk. Kelp has also been shown to reduce oestrogen levels and positively affect the gut microbiome.[40]

Arame: A brown, spaghetti-like sea vegetable with a mild sweet nutty flavour.

Dulse: A red sea vegetable, with a mild smoky flavour, it is considered one of the best-tasting varieties. Dulse can be consumed without the need for soaking because the blades are fairly thin. Has a soft and chewy palatable texture.

Spirulina: Even though spirulina is a plant, the cell walls are primarily protein (not cellulose, as in land plants) which means it is easily digestible. It is a great source of calcium. Make sure the product you buy is freeze-dried as some can be heated to very high temperatures during processing.

Chlorella: This single-celled alga contains all nine essential amino acids. Apart from its incredible nutritional content, chlorella may be able to help reduce oestrogen levels[41] and remove heavy metals as well as other harmful compounds from the body.[42]

Nuts and Seeds

Both are high-energy fuel sources that contain anti-oestrogenic plant sterols and a wide range of essential nutrients. Nuts and seeds should be eaten raw. Roasting alters some of their beneficial qualities, and those commercially packaged are usually cooked in PUFAs and have various chemical preservatives added. Be aware that Brazil nuts, cashews and peanuts are all susceptible to accumulating various mycotoxins and non-organic peanuts are heavily contaminated with pesticides. Always try to store all nuts and seeds in glass containers in the fridge for maximum freshness. Great choices include:

Almonds: Are a wonderful source of vitamin E. Almonds have been shown to improve the gut microbiome[43] as well as significantly decreasing both inflammation and oxidative stress.[44] One problem is that US law demands that all raw almonds be pasteurized or irradiated before being sold. Try to avoid.

Walnuts: Possess potent antioxidant properties, help reduce inflammation and improve the gut microbiome.[45] They are also a substantial source of vitamin E and magnesium.

Pumpkin seeds: Also known as 'pepitas,' these are the edible seeds of a pumpkin. They are flat and oval in shape with a dark green colour. If you're a vegetarian or vegan then pumpkin seeds are an excellent source of zinc, as well as magnesium and manganese.

Hemp seeds: Are the small, dark brown nuts of the hemp plant which are from the same species as cannabis (marijuana). They are exceptionally nutritious but require hulling from their hard shell. Try to source ones that have not been heat sterilized. Hemp seeds don't contain phytic acid, so there is no need for them to be soaked.

Brazil nuts: Are most notable by their antioxidant property, related to their high selenium content. Unfortunately, many Brazil nuts are contaminated with mycotoxins.

Other good choices include pecans, pistachios, macadamias, pine nuts and sunflower seeds. Most nuts and seeds have potent antioxidant properties (usually due to their high vitamin E content), reduce inflammation and can improve the gut microbiome.[45,46]

Nuts and seeds are easier to digest when they have been soaked to neutralize phytic acid and other protective compounds that impede nutrient absorption. Phytic acid is found in other foods including grains and beans. Herbivores such as cows and sheep have the ability to break down this compound but many animals, including humans, cannot. This can be a problem because phytic acid interferes with our ability to absorb important nutrients like zinc, iron, calcium and magnesium. It also inhibits the normal function of digestive enzymes.

Place the raw nuts or seeds in a bowl, cover with pure water (you can also add a sprinkle of sea salt or apple cider vinegar) and set aside to soak. They will plump up as they absorb the water. Brazil nuts, almonds and walnuts contain high amounts of phytic acid and so need to be soaked overnight. Pecans and pistachios contain less so can be soaked for a shorter time. Oily nuts such as macadamia and pine nuts need only an hour or two. To reduce any mycotoxins present you may add some sodium carbonate (not sodium bicarbonate) to the soak water. Next, drain off the water, leave to air-dry in the sun, in an oven on low heat or in a food dehydrator and they are ready to eat. Soaking is also a good way to identify and remove any damaged or spoiled nuts or seeds as they become easier to see.

Fermented Foods and Drinks

These traditional foods have largely disappeared from the Western diet, much to the detriment of our health. Fermentation not only preserves nutrients but also breaks them down into more easily digestible forms as well as making new nutrients. Fermented foods typically contain the antioxidant glutathione, vitamins (particularly B vitamins) and probiotics. They are excellent for your gut microbiome, potent oestrogen detoxifiers as well as having antioxidant, anti-inflammatory and antimicrobial properties.[47] Fermented foods can also help to reduce circulating lipids, blood sugar and insulin levels.[48]

A 2013 study showed that feeding probiotic bacteria to aged mice induced youthful vitality characterised by thick lustrous skin and hair as well as enhanced reproductive health.[49] The researchers showed that the bacteria *Lactobacillus reuteri* increased the growth phase of hair follicles by 106 percent. They proposed this result was caused by reducing the effects of various inflammatory chemicals including TGF-beta1 and TNF. The probiotic bacteria also elevated androgens in the male mice. *L. reuteri* is found in many fermented foods including raw dairy products and sauerkraut.

You can easily make your own or be sure to buy raw fermented foods as most commercial produce is pasteurized and highly filtered. Good choices include sauerkraut, kimchi, apple cider vinegar as well as coconut milk kefir and yoghurt. Check out the informative book *Wild Fermentation: The Flavor, Nutrition, and Craft of Live-Culture Foods* by Sandor Ellix Katz for some ideas. There are also many videos online showing how to make various fermented foods.

Healthy Fats and Oils

"Without enough fat and/or cholesterol the body is severely hampered in its efforts to make steroid hormones, including testosterone." Dr Jonathon V. Wrights

Healthy fat sources are critical for good hormone function. In one study, thirty-nine healthy men between fifty and sixty years were investigated while consuming their usual high fat, low fibre diet.[50] After eight weeks they changed to a low fat, high fibre diet while keeping the same amount of calories. The result of the dietary change was a reduction in total testosterone and free testosterone with an overall 12 percent lowering of circulating androgens. Simply put, a low-fat diet can dramatically decrease your testosterone.

High fat diets correlate with higher levels of testosterone though the type you eat is important. Although all fats and oils, whether animal or plant origin contain a mixture of saturated, monounsaturated and polyunsaturated (PUFA), they differ in their proportion of each.

Saturated fats: These are found mostly in animal products and are solid at room temperature. Good sources include coconut oil, grass-fed butter and ghee as well as grass-fed meat. Saturated fats are needed for calcium to be deposited into bone, protect the liver from alcohol and various medications and help reduce stress. Saturated fats will not increase your risk of heart disease, despite what you may have read.

Researchers in 2014 concluded that: *"Current evidence does not clearly support cardiovascular guidelines that encourage high consumption of polyunsaturated fatty acids and low consumption of total saturated fats."*[51]

In a 2017 review investigators stated: *"Coronary artery disease pathogenesis and treatment urgently requires a paradigm shift. Despite popular belief among doctors and the public, the conceptual model of dietary saturated fat clogging a pipe is just plain wrong. A landmark systematic review and meta-analysis of observational studies showed no association between saturated fat consumption and (1) all-cause mortality, (2) coronary heart disease (CHD), (3) CHD mortality, (4) ischaemic stroke or (5) type 2 diabetes in healthy adults...greater intake of saturated fat was associated with less progression of atherosclerosis whereas carbohydrate and polyunsaturated fat intake were associated with greater progression."*[52]

Dr George V. Mann, scientist in the Framingham Heart Study (one of the longest studies on heart disease), stated: *"The diet-heart hypothesis (that suggests that high intake of fat and cholesterol causes heart disease) has been repeatedly shown to be wrong, and yet, for complicated reasons of pride, profit and prejudice, the hypothesis continues to be exploited by scientists, fund-raising enterprises, food companies, and even governmental agencies. The public is being deceived by the greatest health scam of the century.*"

Monounsaturated fats: Found in olive oil, olives, avocados, nuts and seeds. These fats have been found to be anti-inflammatory,[53] reduce oxidative stress and prevent the release of prostaglandins.[54]

Polyunsaturated fats (PUFAs): Found in vegetable and seed oils, nuts and seeds.

Researchers investigated the consequences of different nutrient factors against their effects on pre-exercise testosterone levels.[55] They found that a diet rich in saturated and monounsaturated raised circulating testosterone but that a diet high in PUFAs decreased levels. Saturated and monounsaturated fats are beneficial for elevating your testosterone and improving your health. Conversely, concentrated PUFAs such as those found in vegetable oil are literally robbing you of your manhood and are detrimental to health.

In general, oils with high smoke points can be cooked at higher temperatures and heating any oil above its smoke point will cause oxidation (rancidity). Oils and fats can oxidize even on the shelf when exposed to oxygen, heat, light and moisture. Therefore, try buying those that are cold-pressed, unrefined and sold in glass bottles. These choices are more expensive than vegetable or seed oils in plastic containers but worth any extra cost. So, which cooking oils are the best to use if you need to avoid all vegetable and seed oils? The following are all recommended:

Coconut Oil: Over 90 percent of the fatty acids in coconut oil are saturated which makes it resistant to heat and so an excellent choice for cooking. This oil is semi-solid at room temperature and can last for years without going rancid. Coconut oil helps lower insulin levels; has antimicrobial, antibacterial and antiviral benefits, as well as being highly anti-inflammatory.[56] Make sure to choose virgin coconut oil, which has been extracted without the application of heat.

Olive Oil: With a unique flavour, olive oil is a great natural source of vitamin E, magnesium and beta-carotene. A relatively low smoke point however, makes it unsuitable for high temperature cooking. Use it on cold dishes or add it only after you have turned off the heat.

Grass-fed Butter and Ghee: Butter is rich in saturated fat and has a medium-low smoke point. Raw organic butter made from grass-fed cow's milk contains the vitamins A, D, E and K_2. However, it is unsuitable for people who are lactose intolerant. Ghee is a type of clarified butter where the milk solids have been removed. This means that casein and lactose, the elements in dairy that many people are sensitive to, are absent. Ghee can also be used at a higher temperature.

Water

An important key to beautiful hair is hydration. Chronic dehydration dries the hair shaft and scalp, ultimately leading to split ends and breakage. As well as this, even a mild dehydrated state leads to increases in cortisol levels. Black tea, coffee and manufactured drinks are not substitutes even though they all contain water.

The amount needed is dependent on many factors including temperature and humidity, activity levels and how much water is taken in through what you eat. It is difficult to make a general recommendation about an intake but the paler your urine is, then the better your state of hydration. Avoid drinking water or fluids with meals as this dilutes the stomach acid and harms digestion. Try drinking from glass bottles and not plastic, as this reduces your exposure to potentially harmful chemicals. Carbon filtered tap water is a good choice.

Herbal Tea

Drinking herbal tea is one of the simplest ways of including beneficial herbs in your daily diet and enjoying their therapeutic benefits, though they are no substitute for healthier eating or a healthy lifestyle. Drinking a hot cup of delicious tea can be a wonderfully relaxing and healing experience in itself. Making a herbal tea (infusion or tisane) is one method of extracting the active and beneficial constituents of an herb. Store-bought tea bags are expensive, lacking in freshness and strength, as well as limited in their variety. Instead, you can find high-quality herbal products in many natural food stores and herb shops, as well as online (see appendix D). You can also pick and grow your own.

It is straightforward to make your own tea from bulk loose herb and the process is not as difficult or time-consuming as you may think. It is better to use fresh rather than dried, whenever possible. Drinking herbal tea provides access to many plants and their nutrients that you wouldn't otherwise consume. It also considerably increases your chance of consuming wild foods that haven't been modified for taste or otherwise altered by man.

There are basically two tea preparations that can be made from loose herbs: an infusion and a decoction. An infusion is made from leaves, flowers and other aerial parts of the plant. A decoction is made if it's the roots or bark being used. All you need for an infusion is a large container (not plastic), tea towel and a strainer. For a decoction, a small stainless steel pot is also required. You will use approximately 200 ml (three-quarters cup) or 300 ml (one and a quarter cup) for a decoction of boiling water for every one heaped teaspoon of herbs.

For an infusion, add the herbs to the container and pour over boiling water. Cover with a damp tea towel and leave to brew for around four hours. Strain and throw away the used herb. It is ready to drink, and you can store the tea in the fridge for three to four days. Add extra water if the tea is too strong or the taste too intense. For a decoction, roots and bark need prolonged heating to extract their nutrients. After you have added the herbs to the pot, pour over boiling water, cover with a lid and gently simmer for fifteen to thirty minutes. Strain, discard the used herb and allow the tea to cool. These can also be stored refrigerated for a number of days.

Herbs must be taken over an extended period of time in order for them to have their desired effects. However, it is best to have intervals of non-use. Drink a couple of cups daily (either hot or cold) but do not add any sugar, artificial sweeteners or milk. Mother Nature is an infinitely better chemist, so my advice is to consume unadulterated natural herbs rather than any man-made concentrated extracts that you may find. Herbs contain hundreds or thousands of active compounds which have a multifaceted effect rather than overwhelming one biochemical pathway and possibly causing side effects. The following are all recommended:

Horny Goat Weed (also known as *epimedium*): According to Chinese folklore the herb was named when farmers noticed their goats became more sexually active after grazing on it. Horny goat weed has demonstrated both antioxidant and anti-inflammatory effects including reducing levels of TNF.[57] It has also been shown to increase free testosterone levels and lower cortisol. This herb contains the active ingredient icariin. In a 2017 animal study icariin promoted hair shaft elongation by prolonging the growth phase while decreasing the resting phase.[58] Another study showed that a high dose of icariin administered to male rats increased their testosterone levels three-fold.[59]

Horsetail: The outer layer of the hair follicle is rich in silica (silicon) and this herb contains the most known in the plant kingdom. This silica is water-soluble, meaning that it can be transported around the body easily. Horsetail has also been shown to have anti-inflammatory properties by reducing the activity of TNF.[60] However, this herb is not recommended for long-term use as it can have adverse effects on the digestive system and inhibit the absorption of vitamin B_1 (thiamine).

Oatstraw: This herb does not contain as much silica as horsetail but it is recommended for long-term use as there are no known negative side effects.

Burdock Root: This fleshy taproot contains inulin, a type of fibre that feeds the good bacteria in your digestive system. Burdock also contains many powerful antioxidants and antidiabetic compounds.[61] The roots are edible raw, cooked or in a decoction or tincture.

Cat's Claw (una de gato): This herb is a tropical vine that grows in the Amazon Rainforest. This vine gets its name from the small thorns at the base of the leaves, which resemble a cat's claw. It has strong anti-viral, antimicrobial, antioxidant and anti-inflammatory properties by suppressing TNF synthesis.[62,63] Cat's claw is an excellent source of the phytonutrient procyanidin B2. It has also demonstrated an incredible ability to cleanse and detoxify the intestinal tract and contributes to restoring a healthier microbiome. This herb can be taken as a decoction or tincture.

Cinnamon: The active principles in this spice are known to have antimicrobial and anti-inflammatory properties while helping to increase enzyme secretions in the digestive system. This herb also helps to regulate blood sugar and prevent insulin resistance.[64] Cinnamon can be used to flavour your meals as well as in herbal decoctions and tinctures. Try using fresh cinnamon stick.

Cloves: This spice has anti-inflammatory properties[65] and improves digestion by increasing enzyme secretions. Cloves are rich in antioxidants and can be used in both decoctions and tinctures. One study showed that one of these antioxidants, eugenol, prevented oxidative damage caused by free radicals five times more effectively than vitamin E, another potent antioxidant.[66]

Cardamom: Part of the ginger family, these small, greenish pods possess antimicrobial and aphrodisiac properties. Nutritionally, no other nutrient in cardamom comes close to the manganese content. Chemicals from cardamom have been shown to lower lipid peroxidation, reduce inflammation by suppressing TNF and minimize oxidative stress by restoring levels of the antioxidant SOD.[67]

Hawthorn: A plant traditionally used to alleviate stress, sleep disorders and pain. The leaves, flowers and berries are all edible and can be used to make tea or tincture. Hawthorn berries have been shown to have both anti-inflammatory and antimicrobial properties.[68] In a 2013 study the effect of a hawthorn berry extract taken orally on hair growth in mice was investigated.[69] The extract promoted the growth phase. The number and the size of hair follicles were also enlarged.

Hibiscus: The flowers and leaves can be used to make a herbal tea and both have antimicrobial, antioxidant and anti-inflammatory properties. Daily consumption has been shown to lower significantly blood pressure and have a positive influence on lipid profiles.[70] In a 2003 study the effects of two hibiscus (*rosa-sinensis*) extracts, one made from leaves and the other from flowers, were tested on rats.[71] They didn't grow any new hairs: however, the leaf extract showed a 25 percent increase in hair length and an elevation in the anagen/telogen ratio. The flower extract showed similar but more modest results.

White Willow Bark: Some of the most useful health benefits include its ability to reduce oxidative stress and inflammation by inhibiting the release of TNF[72] and prostaglandins.[73] This herb can also eliminate pain, soothe the stomach and lower oestrogen levels. The inner bark contains high amounts of salicin (salicylic acid) and can be consumed as a decoction or tincture. Use this herb in moderation and do not take if allergic to aspirin.

Eclipta Prostrata (also known as false daisy or bhringraj): This plant is a member of the sunflower family and the leaves, roots and flowers can be used topically or as a tea. *Eclipta prostrata* has significant antioxidant activity[74] and extracts are known to promote hair growth faster than minoxidil.

In a 2009 study *Eclipta prostrata* applied topically was able to induce the growth phase in 87.5 percent of mice.[75] A 2 percent solution of minoxidil increased the average follicle count from forty-three to seventy-three, whereas *Eclipta prostrata* raised the count from nineteen to sixty-six. In another 2009 study a topical mixture of coconut oil infused with the leaves of *Eclipta prostrata*, flowers of hibiscus (*rosa-sinensis*) and rhizomes of spikenard (*Nardostachys jatamansi*) was shown to promote hair growth in mice.[76] This mixture increased both the growth phase and follicle size significantly more than a 2 percent solution of minoxidil. In a more recent 2015 study *Eclipta prostrata* was shown to stimulate hair growth and reduce the expression of TGF-beta1.[77]

Great Burnet: This hardy herbaceous plant produces spikes of dark red-brown, egg-shaped flowers. The leaves and shoots are used to make tea while the roots, which have the most active constituents, a decoction or tincture. A member of the rose family, this plant possesses anti-inflammatory effects by inhibiting FGF-5, and has been shown to improve hair growth.

In a 2002 study a root extract of great burnet suppressed the conversion of hair follicles from the growth to the resting phase.[78] In a later 2007 study dehaired mice were given a topical extract of great burnet which prolonged the growth phase.[79]

Cacao Shells: These shells are generally considered to be a byproduct of chocolate making. However, they can be used to make a nutritious tea as well as adding flavour to a bitter tasting one. Cacao is one of the best plant-based sources of magnesium and has been shown to have incredible antioxidant properties.[80] You can also eat cacao nibs which are unsweetened pieces of fermented and dried beans.

Tinctures

A tincture is typically an alcoholic extract of plants for use as medicine. The alcohol acts as a solvent, primarily removing the beneficial components from the plants that are water-insoluble. Other solvents can be used such as vinegar or glycerin, though they are less effective. For many herbs, tea is the most effective way to consume them. For other herbs, tinctures are the most useful. The doses with a tincture are much smaller than with teas, the taste factor is less of a problem and they can last for years. If you make your own then use only alcohol for human consumption as your base. Clear vodkas are one of the easiest to use.

How to Make a Tincture
Cut fresh or dried plants/roots into small pieces and place them in a clean glass container. Try not to use a powdered herb for your tinctures. Next, make sure that the alcohol covers the plant material fully. Do not leave any exposed to the air.

Store the jar in a cool, dry, dark place. Shake several times a week and check the alcohol levels. If the alcohol has evaporated and the herb is not totally submerged, be sure to top it up. Herbs exposed to air can introduce mould and bacteria into your tincture. Allow the mixture to steep for six to eight weeks or longer. Then drape a damp piece of cheesecloth (muslin) or unbleached coffee filter over a funnel and pour the contents into another glass container. Discard the used herbs. Label each container and keep in a cool, dark place and your tinctures will last for years. Place what you require into small dropper bottles and use as needed.

You can add some tincture to tea, water or directly into your mouth under the tongue. A trivial amount of alcohol on a daily basis is not harmful to the body. Standard dosage of a tincture is fifteen to forty drops taken three times a day.

Nettle Root: Is the root (rhizome) of the common stinging nettle plant. This herb has been shown to decrease levels of lipid peroxidation,[81] as well as having antioxidant[82] and anti-inflammatory properties by inhibiting the release of prostaglandins.[83] Compounds extracted from nettle root have demonstrated a high affinity for SHBG thus increasing 'free' levels of DHT, testosterone and oestrogen.[84] They have also been shown to possess weak to moderate aromatase-inhibiting effects.[85]

Ashwagandha: Belonging to the same family as the tomato, this herb is an adaptogen popular in Ayurvedic medicine. In one study, after ninety days of men taking five grams daily of ashwagandha powder, significant increases in testosterone and decreases in prolactin were noted, as well as an improvement in the level of antioxidants.[86] This herb has also been shown to raise circulating levels of thyroid hormones in hypothyroid patients,[87] lower cortisol,[88] reduce inflammation and improve sleep quality. Ashwagandha is available in powder and tablet form, as well as the natural root.

He Shou Wu (*polygonum multiflorum* or Fo-Ti [not Fo-ti Tieng]): The name of this herb means 'black-haired Mr. He' in Chinese and refers to a Mr. He who allegedly took the herb and restored his black hair, youthful appearance and vitality. The roots are usually prepared by boiling in a liquid made with black beans. This herb stimulates liver and gall bladder function by increasing bile flow. It also has anti-inflammatory properties[89] and stimulates the production of the antioxidants SOD and glutathione.[90]

A study from 2011 revealed that topical application of He shou wu promoted hair growth by inducing the growth phase in mice.[91] An *in vitro* study from 2013 showed that compounds extracted from this herb increased hair length and promoted a greater development of dermal papilla cells than minoxidil.[92] He shou wu contains emodin which has been revealed to inhibit TGF-beta1 and subsequently reduce fibrosis.[93]

Boswellia (frankincense): This fragrant resin is known for its antimicrobial and anti-inflammatory benefits. It has been demonstrated to be a potent inhibitor of inflammation by preventing TNF activity, both *in vitro* and *in vivo*.[94]

Huanarpo Macho: A shrub-like tree native to Peru. The young branch stems are a popular aphrodisiac and are known to contain high amounts of phytonutrients especially procyanidin B3. The herb has been shown to increase testosterone in mice[95] and can be made into a tincture or decoction.

Mucuna Pruriens (also known as velvet bean): This is a tropical legume native to the Caribbean, Africa and Asia. It is found most commonly in capsule or powdered form, but can also be taken as a tincture. The seeds of the plant contain most of the beneficial bioactive substances. Apart from its nutritional content and adaptogenic properties, this plant has demonstrated several important benefits.

In one study five grams a day of mucuna pruriens seed powder was given to seventy-five infertile men for ninety days. Their levels of testosterone increased whilst prolactin decreased.[96] In another study mucuna pruriens was given to sixty infertile men who were under psychological stress.[97] They took five grams daily of mucuna seed powder for three months. Treatment increased levels of the antioxidants SOD, glutathione and vitamin C, as well as significantly reducing cortisol and the pro-inflammatory chemical lipid peroxide.

FOODS TO AVOID

For almost all of human evolution, we had diets drastically different from the typical Western or Standard American Diet. Many of the foods we eat today are causing inflammation, oxidative stress, lipid peroxidation and upsetting our blood sugar levels. What you eat, as well as the foods you choose not to, is extremely important for the health of the hair. Here are some that should be generally avoided:

Polyunsaturated Fatty Acids (PUFAs)

The single most important product to reduce or eliminate from your diet is concentrated forms of PUFAs. There are two main types of PUFAs: omega-3s and omega-6s. Omega-3s are found naturally in fatty fish, liver and in some nuts and seeds. Omega-6s occur naturally in small quantities in seeds, nuts, legumes as well as grass-fed animal products. By eating moderate amounts of these natural foods we get enough PUFAs in our diet: our fat cells are mostly made from saturated and monounsaturated fat. When consuming PUFAs in concentrated forms, we can end up with a serious imbalance in our bodies and the problems, such as hair loss, that can result.

Although 'vegetable oil' has a healthy sounding name, it's not actually made from vegetables. Most are blends of canola, corn and soybean oils. These as well as seed oils have one major economic advantage: they are cheap. They are found in almost all processed foods and are used for frying in most restaurants and fast-food places. Most of these vegetable and seed oils have a low smoke point making them unsuitable for cooking in the first place. Today the average consumption in the industrialized world is an amazing thirty-two kg (70 lbs) a year. These clear, tasteless, highly refined and processed oils should all be avoided: vegetable, soybean, corn, cottonseed, canola/rapeseed, sesame seed, sunflower, grapeseed, safflower as well as margarine and vegetable shortening. Flax seed, walnut and all fish oils should also be avoided as they are high in concentrated PUFAs. Any animals and their produce that have been fed a diet of corn and soy will also be high in PUFAs.

Vegetable and seed oil have only been used as a food since the turn of the twentieth century. They are usually created with methods that apply extreme heat and pressure, exposing them to all sorts of oxidative damage. Chemicals such as BHA (E320), BHT (E321) and propyl gallate (E310) are added to deodorize and preserve the oil. They are all xenoestrogens. When these oils are repeatedly heated, as they are in restaurants and in the preparation of processed foods, toxic oxidative breakdown products are formed such as formaldehyde (a known human carcinogen) and acrylamide (reduces testosterone levels).[98] Vegetable and seed oils also make an important contribution to mycotoxin exposure as well as containing phytic acid.

As previously discussed, PUFAs can contribute to inflammation, insulin resistance, oxidative damage and lipid peroxidation. There have been many studies revealing their various detrimental effects.

One study showed that when the intake of saturated and monounsaturated fats was raised testosterone subsequently increased but when the consumption of PUFAs was elevated, testosterone significantly decreased.[99]

In one review researchers noted several aspects of these oils: increased production of prostaglandins and TNF (both inflammatory markers), as well as promotion of the activity of the aromatase enzyme.[100]

In another review it was shown that the type of fat consumed directly influences thyroid activity: saturated fats improved thyroid function while PUFAs decreased performance.[101]

Another study revealed Israel has one of the highest consumptions of omega-6 PUFA in the world. This country also has a prevalence of cardiovascular disease, hypertension, type 2 diabetes and insulin resistance. The researchers concluded these problems were directly owing to their high omega-6 PUFA diets.[102]

Lastly, in one paper the lead researcher argues the main cause of heart disease is not dietary cholesterol but rather oxidized (damaged) cholesterol and fats. *"Vegetables oils, partially hydrogenated fats, and fried foods are responsible for the persistently high rate of heart disease. The most effective way to prevent coronary heart disease and sudden death according to these conclusions is to eat fewer commercially fried foods, fewer polyunsaturated fats and to avoid partially hydrogenated fats. Conversely, we should eat more vegetables and fruit as a source of antioxidants."*[103]

Avoiding them however is easier said than done as their presence is insidious in our food supply. They are present in almost all processed foods as well as most restaurant and fast-food. To avoid them, start preparing as many of your meals as possible at home using healthier cooking oils, such as coconut oil.

Refined Grains

Our ancestors ate grains as well as fruit in their whole and unprocessed state. However, our diets today include a high percentage of refined carbohydrates. The average American now eats ten servings of refined grains each day, mostly wheat in the form of white flour. If nothing else, consuming such large amounts displaces more nutritious foods. The processing of carbohydrates makes these foods more readily absorbable, causing problems for our insulin and fat metabolism. This, in turn, contributes to altered circulating lipids, insulin resistance and type 2 diabetes. In addition, they are known to increase levels of inflammation.[104] Refined grains are also a significant source of phytic acid and mycotoxin exposure.

For these reasons, refined grains should be avoided, especially enriched bleached white flour found in most bread, pastries, pasta, crackers and cookies. If you want to eat bread, do not go for whole grain but rather a quality rye sourdough or sprouted bread. Sourdough is made by the fermentation of dough which partially breaks down gluten and is usually easier to digest than regular bread. The process of sprouting (germinating) grains before they're ground into flour minimizes phytic acid, mycotoxins and other substances to which some people may be sensitive or allergic.

The answer is not to stop eating carbohydrates completely, just those that have been refined and processed. Glucose is the major fuel for hair follicles and a steady supply is needed for optimal growth. Inadequate carbohydrate intake has also been shown to decrease testosterone while increasing cortisol levels.[105] Carbohydrates are essential for the conversion of thyroid hormone to its active form and help to remove excess oestrogen from the body.

It is, however, important to soak all grains in water, just as you should nuts and seeds. Soaking grains has many positive benefits including reducing gluten and other anti-nutrients, mycotoxins, pesticides and any toxins present. This is especially important for rice which has around ten to twenty times more arsenic than other cereal crops. Soaking quinoa reduces saponin content which not only gives this grain a bitter taste but can also irritate the gut. Like nuts, most grains contain phytic acid that binds to crucial minerals such as calcium, magnesium, copper, iron and especially zinc in the digestive tract, making them more difficult to absorb. Regular consumption of untreated whole grain can potentially lead to depletion of these vital nutrients.

Soaking grains in warm water reduces phytic acid as well as other anti-nutrients such as lectins. You can also add a small amount of an acidic liquid, such as apple cider vinegar or lemon juice, to aid this process. To reduce any mycotoxins present you can add some sodium carbonate (not sodium bicarbonate). Buckwheat, brown rice and millet have low levels of phytic acid and require around seven hours soaking. All other grains should be left overnight for at least twelve hours.

Sugars, High-Fructose Corn Syrup and Soda

Why we eat so much sugar is not difficult to understand. The problem is that most people don't realise quite how much they consume. The average adult in America now eats twenty to thirty teaspoons every day or about seventy-seven kg (170 lbs) per year. A diet this high in added sugar can induce changes in the gut including increases in oestrogen, endotoxins and inflammation.[106] It can also decrease your thyroid function and lower antioxidant levels.

Traditional Chinese medicine believes immoderate consumption of sugar is the main culprit responsible for hair loss. Sometimes we know we're eating sugar but often we don't. Processed foods and drinks are the biggest sources of added sugar with around 75 percent of all packaged foods and beverages in the US containing them.

The worst of these sweeteners is probably high-fructose corn syrup (HFCS). If you see this sweetener on a label, the food is probably processed junk. It contains no enzymes, vitamins or minerals. HFCS causes problems with the digestive system, decreases insulin sensitivity[107] and is frequently contaminated with mercury. Avoid all products with this ingredient especially soda (soft drinks).

According to a study by *Yale University*, the average American consumes 170 litres (forty-five gallons) of sugary, sweetened beverages a year.[108] As these are averages, it means many people are consuming far greater amounts. Apart from sugar and HFCS, soda can contain phosphoric acid and artificial sweeteners such as aspartame. It has also been shown that: "S*SB* [sugar-sweetened beverage] *consumption is significantly associated with low serum testosterone in men 20 to 39 years old in the United States.*"[109] Consuming SSBs also leads to an increase in inflammatory markers, insulin resistance and circulating lipids.[110] People who drink soda are also far more likely to be deficient in vitamin A, calcium and magnesium. One reason is the phosphoric acid (phosphorus) content that interferes with the body's ability to absorb these nutrients. This contributes significantly toward calcification.

There are also problems with artificial sweeteners. Products that are labelled 'low calorie,' 'diet' or 'no sugar added' are likely to contain them. These include aspartame (Equal, NutraSweet, E951), saccharin (Sweet 'N Low) and sucralose (Splenda). These sweeteners have been demonstrated to produce endotoxins and negatively affect the microbiome as well as contributing to metabolic syndrome and type 2 diabetes.[111] Splenda has been shown to reduce the amount of good bacteria in the intestines by 50 percent.[112] The FDA (US Food and Drug Administration) listed ninety-two adverse reactions associated with the sweetener aspartame: hair loss, thinning and baldness were all included.

Sometimes it is not so much the sugar content that is the problem but the food will also contain refined wheat, PUFAs and various other sweeteners and chemicals. If you do have a sweet tooth, then stevia is one option. Eating more fresh fruit is also a good idea. Good quality dark chocolate (72 percent cacao or greater) without any additives such as soy lecithin is another alternative. I believe an effective way to eliminate a craving for refined sugars is to start consuming bitter and sour foods and herbs. This has a profound effect over time, adjusting our taste buds away from the excessive sweet and salty flavours of processed food. Over time this will reduce cravings for packaged foods and refined sugars.

Processed Food

"How pathetically little we really know about processed food, the food that sits on supermarket shelves in boxes, cartons and bottles, everything that comes wrapped or packed in some way, food that has had something done to it to make it more convenient and read-to-eat." Joanna Blythman, *Swallow This*

Processed foods are, more or less, 60 to 70 percent of what most men in the US and the UK eat today. It is convenient and insidious in our society. In a short period of time, we have digressed from an almost totally natural diet to one full of food colourings: artificial flavours and sweeteners; pesticides and other biocides; processed soy; refined carbohydrates; PUFAs; thickeners; glazing agents; synthetic hormones and, most recently, genetically engineered foods. Over three thousand chemicals are added to our food supply as well as more than ten thousand solvents, emulsifiers and preservatives.

Processed foods often contain various man-made chemicals that have known deleterious effects. In the small amounts that are present, we have been assured that there is no need for concern as they will not negatively impact our health. Admittedly there are only minute amounts of these additives in each portion of processed food you eat. But it all adds up, with the average American consuming around four and a half kg (ten lbs) of chemical additives a year. The combined cocktail effects of all these chemicals have not been tested. There are many different factors that negatively impact our health. Therefore, it is difficult to predict how a certain artificial sweetener such as aspartame or preservative like sodium benzoate will increase our risk, for example, of hair loss after consuming it for ten years. We really don't know what effect continuous amounts of these chemicals will have over many years.

In the further words of Joanna Blythman: "*Researchers observe what dose laboratory animals can take of a substance before showing obvious signs of illness, or dying, and then extrapolate from this the likely effects on humans. But this is an informed estimate; no one really knows how much of a carcinogen it takes to cause cancer, or how much of a toxin it takes to poison your nervous system.*"

Processed foods use antimicrobial preservatives to kill bacteria that cause food to spoil. These compounds work like antibiotics: they kill microbes in the products but they can also destroy the good bacteria within your gut. The more we traumatize our microbiome, the more we are likely to suffer from chronic inflammation. Some common antimicrobial preservatives are also xenoestrogens. With so many additives to avoid, the simplest strategy is to focus on eating whole, fresh and unprocessed foods.

The closer a food is to its natural state the better. Every item you see listed on an ingredient label should be readily understandable and familiar. Use your common sense. Many foods come with an abundance of nutrition labels but this is mostly a confusing waste of time. Companies spend billions of dollars every year aggressively promoting their products, despite them degrading your quality of health. The most effective way to avoid all these various additives is to cook and eat food from scratch in your own home, even if you don't consider yourself a great chef. Admittedly, cooking takes more time and is far less convenient but considering the huge benefits, it doesn't take that much time or effort.

Grain-fed Animal Protein

"Recent studies indicate that of all the toxic chemical residues in the American diet, almost all, 95% to 99%, comes from meat, fish, dairy products and eggs." John Robbins, *Diet For a New America*

Hair is primarily made of protein and, therefore, it makes sense to have a protein-rich diet if you're trying to maintain healthy growth. The issue is not that eating meat itself is bad for your health but that the quantity and quality that most men eat today is a serious problem. The average American consumes around eighty-five kg (186 lbs) annually, most of it muscle meat and from grain-fed animals.

Embedded into our cultural fabric is the connection between meat and protein, although there's plenty in the plant world. Many of the largest, most muscular animals on Earth are vegetarians. Plant foods have every essential amino acid and we do not need to seek out protein from concentrated animal sources to make sure we are getting enough.

Eating meat is also associated with masculinity. For men in many parts of the world, it's not a meal unless it contains meat. There is a common assumption that vegetarians (and vegans especially), must have lower testosterone than their carnivorous counterparts. Researchers have directly compared testosterone levels in vegans, vegetarians and meat-eaters.[113] Vegetarians and meat-eaters had virtually equal levels and vegans were higher by about 6 percent. However, there were no differences between the diet groups in their levels of free testosterone.

Meat is therefore unnecessary for healthy testosterone production. Conversely, many studies have shown that men who switch from meat-based to plant-based diets do experience a reduction in their testosterone. On plant-based diets, many men tend to eat very little saturated fat and too much PUFA, soy and refined carbohydrates, all of which negatively affect their levels.

If you eat animal produce then always try to purchase 'hormone-free.' This is important as steroid hormones are injected to fatten commercially raised animals and man-made oestrogens mixed into their feed. These are stored in their fat and muscle fibres and are passed into their produce. It is also estimated that more than 90 percent of the pesticides Americans consume are found in the fat and tissue of meat and dairy products.

There is a huge difference between well-reared, organic grass-fed meat and that which is factory farmed. Many of the health problems associated with eating beef are really with corn, soy or grain-fed beef. Cows are natural herbivores and are healthiest when they eat grass, rather than the unnatural diet they are fed in confinement meat and dairy operations. For these reasons, only consume meat that has been pasture-fed, labelled as being hormone-free and preferably organic. For more information about pasture-based farming, check out the website: www.eatwild.com.

In his informative book *Missing Microbes: How the Overuse of Antibiotics is Fueling our Modern Plagues* author and infectious-disease expert Martin J. Blaser says: "*...antibiotic resistance is not just a problem of people overusing antibiotics. The problem also stems from how we treat animals down on the farm. Today, an estimated 70–80 percent of all antibiotics sold in the United States are used for the single purpose of fattening up farm animals.*"

These issues also apply to poultry and their eggs. Chickens are raised in crowded pens, under artificial light both night and day and fed substandard food as well as antibiotics. Conventionally raised chickens often have elevated levels of arsenic owing to the drugs and chemicals used in their production. Their eggs are inferior in nutritional qualities to those of properly nourished hens.[114] Buy hormone-free, organic eggs whenever available. The label 'free-range' is essentially meaningless.

This doesn't mean you need to eliminate meat from your diet, just be careful of the quality and quantity that you consume. Unfortunately, a lot of men eat meat as part of two or even three meals a day, almost exclusively muscle meat. Learn to eat the organs of animals such as the liver, while home-made bone broth is another great choice.

Animals from the sea, like sustainable varieties of fish, are preferable to land animals: but avoid all farmed fish. These are also subject to many of the same issues as land animals, namely high antibiotic and pesticide use, as well as genetically modified feed. One report warned that farmed salmon contained ten times the number of toxins of wild salmon.[115]

Unfortunately fish, both wild and farmed, can be some of the most polluted foods we eat: often contaminated with toxins such as mercury and PCBs. Mercury is highly toxic, and exposure for many people is large fish, tuna being the single most common source. The oils made from farmed fish are also highly contaminated. Avoid tuna along with bluefish, sea bass, marlin, mackerel, shark, swordfish, Atlantic or farmed salmon, perch, grouper and all shellfish, as these are commonly the most polluted varieties. Safer seafood choices include wild Alaskan salmon, sardines, anchovies, sole, haddock, Atlantic herring, Pacific cod and trout. For more information check this website: www.seafoodwatch.org.

Industrial Dairy

Modern industrial milk and other dairy products are generally from animals raised indoors and fed on corn, grain or soybeans, all of which are unnatural for herbivores to eat. Dairy cows are also treated with powerful antibiotics including penicillin, as well as a range of growth hormones. All commercial dairy products are pasteurized, meaning they are heated to extremely high temperatures to kill any potential bacteria. This processing reduces the nutritional quality and kills enzymes that are required to absorb the fat, lactose and calcium. There is no reason to eat modern industrial dairy, and there are numerous studies on its detrimental effects.[116]

In one study researchers examined the sex hormones in men after they had drunk commercial cow's milk.[117] After drinking only 600 ml, their levels of oestrogen significantly increased followed by a significant decrease in testosterone. This happened within one hour. Researchers have also shown cow's milk can contain up to twenty chemicals including painkillers, antibiotics, growth hormones, triclosan (xenoestrogen) as well as oestrogen.[118] One of the most common food allergies is cow's milk, which also contains high levels of phosphorus.

Try sourcing raw milk that is full-fat, non-homogenized, hormone-free and from grass-fed animals. Full-fat milk enables the body to absorb the protein and calcium. Raw milk also tastes much better though it should be consumed within a few days of purchase. Soured and fermented raw products such as kefir are also great for your digestive system. Commercial 'probiotic' yoghurts, however, are not recommended.

A good substitute is unsweetened almond milk: not only is it high in vitamin E but also it's delicious and tastes like regular milk. Hemp and coconut milk are other good choices.

Flax and Soy

Flax and flax oil have the image of being super healthy. Forget its omega-3 content, it is the number one phytoestrogen containing food. Flax is the richest source of lignan, having levels 800-fold over that of most other foods.[119] Lignan has been shown to decrease total and free testosterone levels.

In one case study a thirty-one-year-old woman ate thirty grams a day of flax for four months.[120] Her total testosterone dropped by 70 percent and free testosterone by 89 percent. Admittedly, the study was on one woman but the decrease is staggering with the sole purpose being to reduce her testosterone and excess hair growth using flax. Researchers also looked at forty male subjects who took thirty grams (two tablespoons) of flax a day for a month. Their total testosterone decreased by around 10 percent.[121]

Although considered the perfect alternative to meat by many, processed soy is the second highest phytoestrogens-containing food. It is also heavily contaminated with pesticides and the toxic metal cadmium, as well as being by far the biggest potential dietary source of the known toxin hexane. Soy also contains the highest levels of phytic acid of any grain or legume. Up to 80 percent of the oil we consume today is soybean. Since it is a cheap form of protein, soy is now found in around two-thirds of all processed food. Like flax, unlabelled genetically modified soybeans are common.

Processed soy can lead to male hormonal and fertility problems, as well as negatively affecting thyroid function.[122] In one study twelve men (mean age just over thirty-two) consumed fifty-six grams of pure soy protein powder daily for twenty-eight days.[123] Their total serum testosterone decreased by 19 percent. In another study, the effects of replacing meat in the diet with a soy product (tofu) on forty-two healthy men aged thirty-five to sixty-two were evaluated. Overall androgen activity decreased and the ratio of testosterone/oestrogen was found to be significantly lower in those men eating tofu.[124]

Tofu, soy milk, soy burgers and other processed products containing soy protein isolates or concentrate should be avoided. Conversely, fermented organic soy in such products as tempeh, miso or natto is much lower in phytoestrogens and phytic acid. They are also an excellent source of vitamin K_2.

Part 5: Good Hair Care

TOPICAL SOLUTIONS

Men use an average of six personal-care products a day, with each of these containing about twelve chemicals. We are literally washing, spraying and covering ourselves with dozens of chemicals every single day of the year. While many of these are harmless, some are known carcinogens, neurotoxins or mimic oestrogen in the body. Unlike the food we eat, these compounds are not processed by the liver to remove any toxic substances that may be present.

There is a constant exchange between your body and its environment, with some substances we put on our skin being directly absorbed into our bloodstream and lymphatic system. Our skin, including our scalps, protects us from exposure to certain chemicals while intensifying the effects of others. It does a good job at keeping out water and large proteins but substances like fat and hormones, including xenoestrogens, are readily absorbed. Absorption rates (when the chemical actually makes it into the bloodstream) on our face and scalp are five to ten times higher than on other parts of our body.

Overall, healthy hair is not only about the visible shaft; but also the follicle, sebaceous gland and the general well-being of the skin where the hair is rooted. Dandruff and a history of skin disease are both associated with hair loss.[1] For a healthy scalp you need to remove regularly all dead skin, accumulated toxins, product residue and old sebum. New growth cannot push its way out of the scalp if it is blocked at all. According to an article in the British newspaper *The Telegraph*: many shampoos contain ingredients that deposit product on the skin, and therefore have a cumulatively damaging effect on the health of the scalp.[2] Cosmetic chemist Dr Joe Cincotta states: "...*the new, soft hair can't push through the build-up on the scalp. This damage is sometimes irreversible.*"

Shampoo, Conditioners and Personal-Care Products

The cuticle is the outer protective layer of each individual hair. It is rich in silicon and minimizes the movement of moisture in and out of the shaft. However, application of chemical products you may use for cleaning, conditioning or styling as well as weathering, can weaken the integrity of this layer and disrupt this balance. When the cuticle is damaged, your hair is more prone to breakage and splitting. In contrast, when your cuticles are healthy, they protect the inner layers from damage and improve overall appearance.

Shampoo cleans the scalp and hair by loosening dirt and oils. Conditioners prevent tangling and protect the hair from drying out and becoming too brittle. When it comes to their hair, a lot of men just slap on any product and hope for the best. It is such an accepted part of modern life that you might not ever have read the ingredients list on any bottle, despite the fact that most commercially available ones today use harmful and potentially carcinogenic ingredients. These dangerous chemicals are also likely to be found in many so-called hair loss products.

If your shampoo or conditioner has any of the following listed toxic chemicals (and they probably do), then throw them in the bin. It's time to change. Many of the ingredients are chemical creations from petroleum and companies don't have to list all the materials in their products, so you don't even know what you are putting on your body. At the end of the day your health is your personal responsibility, not the government's nor your doctor's and certainly not any companies. We have to look to ourselves to find out what is safe and what to avoid.

Limit yourself to those products you really need, and give your body a break from the barrage of chemicals it has to deal with on a daily basis. We don't really know what the risks are for the majority of chemicals found in consumer products. Whilst labels can make all kinds of claims on the front of the bottle, it is the fine print on the back that you need to pay close attention to. Don't be misled by words such as 'natural,' 'herbal' or 'organic.' While you are at it, check all products in your bathroom including sunscreen, toothpaste, deodorant, hair dye, aftershave, lip balms, mouthwash, cough syrups and even household cleaning items for the following chemicals.

7 Chemicals to Strictly Avoid

Sodium Lauryl Sulfate (SLS) & Sodium Laureth Sulfate (SLES): SLS is used in testing laboratories as the standard ingredient to irritate skin. Both SLS and SLES are xenoestrogens and are used widely as major ingredients in cosmetics, toothpaste, conditioner and shampoos because they are cheap. Sulfates are found in more than 90 percent of shampoos and body washes. Most products with the hair loss medication minoxidil also contain SLS.

Researchers have stated that: *"...surfactants such as sodium lauryl sulfate (SLS) in shampoos can penetrate easily into the structure of hair...leading to loosening of hair in the follicular cavity, ultimately leading to hair loss."*[3] Put differently, one of the most common ingredients in shampoos has been shown to cause hair loss.

According to the American College of Toxicology, any concentration above 2 percent SLS will cause some degree of irritation to your skin.[4] This susceptibility increases with ingredient concentration, although this irritation may or may not be evident to the user. Most shampoos are around 15 percent concentration. The National Toxic Encephalopathy Foundation has stated that deposits of SLS can slow hair growth and lead to hair loss. SLS is also capable of stripping away too much sebum, resulting in a very dry and irritated scalp. So, can your shampoo actually contribute to your hair loss? Yes, it can.

There are milder versions of SLS and other surfactants made from coconut oil such as coco betaine but they are still detergents. To be truly safe, steer clear of all detergents in shampoo entirely.

Selenium Sulfide: This is a chemical found in many dandruff shampoos and treatments including some well-known products such as Head and Shoulders and Selsun. Selenium sulfide has a few known side effects including: hair loss, hair discolouration and excessive dryness or oiliness of the scalp/hair. It is also probably a human carcinogen.[5]

Parabens (E214, E215, E218, E219): These chemicals are preservatives to prevent bacteria from growing, and are found in many skincare products including shampoo. Most have the word paraben in their name but they can also be listed as benzoates. They cause a weak oestrogen effect on the body (they are xenoestrogens) and easily penetrate the skin. Researchers have stated that parabens from topical application can reduce your testosterone levels.[6]

Phthalates: These controversial chemicals control viscosity and stop products from separating. They can take on many names making it more difficult to identify (if listed at all.) Check the ingredient label for words ending in phthalate or DEP, DBP and DEHP. Phthalates are xenoestrogens and are absorbed through the skin (refer to part 6 for more information on their detrimental effects).

Fragrance: While sounding very pleasant, 'fragrance' (or parfum) is a euphemism for nearly four thousand different chemicals. Many of these synthetic ingredients are recognised hormone disruptors and xenoestrogens, or otherwise toxic. According to the *Environmental Working Group*, 75 percent of products that list fragrance among their ingredients contain phthalates.

Formaldehyde: This chemical is a toxin, allergen and carcinogen. It is frequently found as a contaminant that enters a product by way of antimicrobial preservatives called formaldehyde-releasers, which release the chemical over time. The most common of these include quaternium-15, diazolidinyl urea, imidazolidinly urea and DMDM hydantoin. They are one of the main causes of allergic contact dermatitis; a known cause of hair loss.[7] It is unclear how formaldehyde affects our bodies when it is absorbed through our skin as there is not enough research available.

Triclosan: An antibacterial agent that's often added to personal-care products such as: shampoo, soaps, deodorants, mouth washes and toothpaste as a preservative. Triclosan is a known endocrine disruptor (xenoestrogen) especially of thyroid and reproductive hormones.[8] It is also a skin irritant and almost certainly disrupts our microbiome. The US has recently banned several antimicrobial chemicals, including triclosan, but the restriction only applied to soaps, not toothpaste nor shampoo.

For more information about the toxicity of specific products and ingredients, check this website: www.safecosmetics.org.

Home-made Shampoo and Conditioner

You should never forget that the oils (sebum) that your hair needs are naturally produced on the scalp. Cleaning hair strips these protective oils along with any dirt, possibly leading to excessive production. Although it may sound counterintuitive, washing your hair too often can actually make it greasy. Men with hair loss have been shown to have increased sebum production[9] and there are several possible explanations for this including: stress, hormonal imbalances, nutritional deficiency (especially vitamins B_2 and B_6), washing with water that is too hot and overuse of incorrect hair products.

Especially after exercise or even just another day in the city, most men like to wash the grime and sweat from their hair. Understandable though this is, one to two times a week should be enough, even with 100 percent natural products. Sebum cannot be replenished if we wash our hair too often. The cold and dry air in winter as well as air-conditioned interiors can also contribute to this problem. Many men shampoo their hair repeatedly with commercial products that contribute to not only excess sebum production but also product build-up on the scalp.

It's okay not to buy regular shampoo or conditioner, as there are many simple home-made ways to clean your hair and scalp. What will work for you depends on your hair texture, density and porosity as well as its length and colour. Initially, there may be a difficult period of adjustment before positive effects start to show. Your hair will then start producing its natural oils at a slower rate. While you may make some compromises along the way, it's not about using things that don't work. These alternatives will give you the same or similar results just without the toxic chemicals. Shampoos didn't exist until the 1930s. Before its advent, most people didn't roam the streets with dirty greasy heads. Rather, they had already identified how to clean their hair using natural things available around them. Any products we use should nourish and strengthen, rather than just clean or make it look good.

I understand that the idea of making your own shampoo and conditioner is somewhat strange to many men. It is one of those modern-day conveniences we just take for granted but preparing your own doesn't take long and the following ones are all very easy and cheap to make. Natural ingredients have healing powers that simply cannot be recreated by synthetic creations. There is no reason to rely on chemicals to make a product work or even to preserve it. However, if one of your home-made products begins to smell bad, throw it out. If the idea of making your own is too extreme, then there are plenty of natural shampoos and conditioners on the market that use plant derived ingredients in place of harsh and dangerous chemicals. There are numerous brands out there including Aubrey Organics, Morrocco Method and many others.

Natural Shampoo: You will need 250 ml (one cup) of distilled water, two tablespoons of herbs (such as calendula, chamomile, sage, nettle leaf, thyme or rosemary), six tablespoons of liquid castile soap (Dr. Bronner's is a good brand) and a quarter teaspoon of jojoba oil. Begin by boiling the water. Add the herbs and let simmer for around fifteen to twenty minutes. Strain and cool. Discard the used herbs. Slowly add the castile soap and then mix in the jojoba oil. Shake before using.

Clay: The topical use of clay for cleaning the skin and hair can be traced throughout ancient history. You may feel your skin is tingling and 'alive' as it has an amazing ability to absorb toxins and impurities. A clay mask can clean the shafts and remove any excess sebum, dead skin or product residue on the scalp.

The rough proportions are going to be one part clay to two parts warm water: enough to make a thick paste. You can also use a herbal infusion instead of water for your preparation. Other variations are to mix ground cinnamon, amla (Indian gooseberry) powder or eclipta prostrata powder in with the clay. The mixture tends to stay lumpy, so it usually takes a few minutes to mix thoroughly. Spread the mask on your hair and scalp, and leave for around twenty minutes. Wash the mask off with warm water. If you have normal/dry hair then choose French green, bentonite or kaolin (white) clay. If you have oily hair then choose rhassoul (red) clay. Afterward, as it dries out the hair and scalp, apply some fresh aloe vera or a herbal infusion.

Soda and Vinegar Hair Cleanser: Baking soda (not baking powder) or bicarbonate of soda is an inexpensive option to clean your hair and scalp. This is known as a fantastic cleaning product in general. It's a mild alkali with fine, slightly abrasive particles. These two factors work together to effectively break down dirt and grease, which can then be easily rinsed away. Apple cider vinegar (ACV) has antibacterial and antifungal properties that help heal an itchy, dry scalp. It is a natural conditioner and can improve your hair's ability to absorb and maintain moisture. This can make each strand shinier, stronger and less prone to breakage and tangling. An ACV rinse also balances the alkalinity of baking soda.

First mix together one teaspoon of baking soda and 100 ml of hot water and stir until fully dissolved. Let cool and it's ready to use. Then take 50 ml of ACV and mix with 50 ml water. Don't use white vinegar: it's too acidic. Like many natural cleaners, this isn't a one-size-fits-all recipe; it should be adjusted to suit your needs. Men with oily hair might require a bit more baking soda. After wetting your hair, pour the soda mixture over your head little by little. Massage it into your scalp, focusing on the roots. Leave it for three to four minutes, then rinse well. Repeat the process with the vinegar wash, being careful not to get it into your eyes or on your face. Once again, rinse well. You may have a slight vinegar smell immediately after your shower but this will fade away quickly. Don't do it too often, however, as it will dry out your hair, so leave a few days between washes.

Aloe Vera: The leaves of this cactus-looking plant hold a translucent gel that brings a refreshing and cooling sensation when applied to the scalp. It helps to remove dead skin cells, prevents bacterial and fungal infections, heals irritated skin and leaves the hair soft and silky. It is a great natural moisturizer and conditioner: protecting the hair and the body from the sun and other harsh weather conditions.

As a shampoo: Mix the gel of a two-inch piece with half a teaspoon of sea salt and half a teaspoon of baking soda in a blender. Gently rub this mixture into the scalp for a few minutes and then rinse out.

As a conditioner: Use following a shower, after having washed your hair or spent time in the sun. Cut a two to three inch piece of leaf, trim off the spikes and slice down the middle. Gently massage the gel on to your hair and scalp. You can use as often as you like.

Instead of buying hair products containing this ingredient from the market, purchase fresh aloe leaves or even better still, grow your own. Aloe vera is very low maintenance, so see if you can grow a few of these amazing plants in your home or garden.

Herbal Rinses

Herbal infusions can penetrate the hair shaft giving the active ingredients a chance to nourish and enrich your natural hair colour. They can also be quite therapeutic for the scalp and help relieve dryness and itchiness. Herbal rinses are especially good for men who are frequent exercisers, as they help to wash out sweat and dirt while adding nutrients. Herbal hair rinses are 100 percent natural, very simple and cheap to make. Some of the recommended nourishing herbs you can use are rosemary, nettle leaf, chamomile and nasturtium. Feel free to be creative and experiment to find what herbs work for your hair.

Method: Create a herbal infusion by pouring 250 ml (one cup) of boiling water over two or three teaspoons of herbs of your choice. Allow to steep for at least an hour in a stainless steel or glass container (not plastic nor aluminium) and keep covered. Strain the infusion, and it's ready to use. It's that simple. Pour the rinse slowly over your hair after a shower. If you can, catch the drippings into another bowl and keep on pouring them through your hair. Massage the infusion into your scalp and either rinse out with cool water or, if you prefer, just leave it on. Your infusion can be stored in the fridge for a few days if there is any left over. You can use as often as you like.

Rosemary: This aromatic herb is beneficial for helping hair grow when used topically. Rosemary cleanses the scalp as it has excellent anti-inflammatory, anti-bacterial and anti-fungal properties, helping to fight microbe infections, lice and other harmful organisms. Rosemary can also improve circulation and promote new cell growth on the scalp.

Nettle leaf: Stinging nettle leaf conditions your hair, helps with dandruff or an irritated scalp, as well as reducing inflammation. This herb is particularly good for men with oily hair.

Chamomile: With its anti-inflammatory, anti-irritant and antimicrobial properties, this herb is highly effective in preventing dandruff and soothing an itching scalp.

Nasturtium: This plant has strong antimicrobial and anti-inflammatory properties. The leaves and orange, red, purple or yellow flowers can be used to make a tea or herbal rinse. The leaves and flowers are also edible. Ancient South Americans used nasturtium to promote hair growth.

Alternative method: Instead of just using water, you can also add raw apple cider vinegar (ACV). Pour around 500 ml (two cups) of ACV in a glass jar and add five to ten teaspoons of fresh herbs. Make sure the herbs are fully covered. Let this sit for at least two weeks. You can then store in the fridge where it will last for several months. When you want to use, dilute a tablespoon of the infused ACV with 250 ml (one cup) of water and apply like a water infusion. Be careful not to get into your eyes.

Oils

One popular method to stimulate hair growth throughout history has been to use oils. They are lubricants and sealants that can trap moisture in the hair and prevent its depletion. However, using oil alone as a moisturizer will only cause dryness over a period of time. They are best used as a leave-in, applied to damp hair or before going into a sauna or steam room. How much to apply is a matter of personal preference, though a little generally goes a long way.

Oily skin and hair are the result of overactive sebaceous glands. Not only does this look unsightly, it can be the starting point of problems such as seborrheic dermatitis (seborrhea), dandruff and hair loss. It may seem counterintuitive to use oil on oily hair and skin but surprisingly they can help reduce oiliness by regulating sebum production. Researchers have also found that: *"Oils play an important role in protecting hair from damage...Applying oil on a regular basis can enhance lubrication of the shaft and help prevent hair breakage.*"[10]

All oils should preferably be cold-pressed and stored in glass. Cold pressing ensures that the maximum possible amount of oil's character and nutritional content are preserved. 'Cold filtered' is not necessarily the same. Three of the best choices you can use are:

Castor Oil: This odourless oil has been used for centuries to treat scalp irritation and stimulate hair growth. It contains high amounts of ricinoleic acid which has anti-inflammatory, antimicrobial and antioxidant properties, protecting the scalp from microbial and fungal infections. This oil contains high levels of the natural antioxidant vitamin E and applied topically has also been shown to reduce the effects of PGD_2- a known inhibitor of hair growth.[11] Castor oil is good to mix with another oil as it tends to be too thick on its own.

Jojoba Oil: Obtained from the fragrant seeds of the jojoba plant, it's not actually oil but rather a liquid wax and so has no rancidity factor, as oils do. This odourless, golden-coloured wax closely resembles sebum and has antimicrobial and anti-inflammatory activity, mediated through the decrease of TNF.[12] Jojoba oil has a very low melting point, so remains in the liquid state and also doesn't have as much of a greasy feel as oils.

Coconut Oil: This oil's antibacterial and antifungal properties protect your scalp against dandruff and lice, both of which can hinder hair growth. Coconut oil penetrates deep inside the hair shaft,[13] exhibits anti-inflammatory properties and also smells good. If you are using coconut oil which is in a solid or semi-solid state, place the jar in hot water until it turns to liquid.

Hair oil can also act as a medium to supply nutrients to the scalp and hair follicles when infused with herbs. To do this you take four tablespoons (quarter cup) of herbs along with 250 ml (one cup) of carrier oil. Place this mixture in a large bowl over a boiling pan of water and warm for at least ten minutes on very low heat. Let it cool, strain the infused oil, discard any herb and pour into a glass airtight container. If the products separate between uses, simply shake the mixture. Infused oils can last for years if stored properly.

Topical use of rosemary oil has been shown to increase blood flow in the scalp, improve hair growth and inhibit 5-alpha reductase (reducing DHT levels).[14] In a 2015 study of 100 patients with MPB, no significant difference was found between rosemary oil applied daily and a 2 percent minoxidil topical.[15] No notable changes were observed after three months but both groups demonstrated a significant increase in hair count after six months. The most common adverse effect reported was scalp itching, more frequent with minoxidil use. Something as simple as applying oil infused with rosemary on the scalp can be as efficacious as the most popular hair-loss medication.

In a 2017 study, a topical treatment of Siberian geranium (*Geranium sibiricum*) promoted more significant hair growth in mice and development of human dermal papilla cells than minoxidil.[16] The researchers concluded Siberian geranium possibly inhibited TGF-beta1 activity. The ability of this plant to affect hair growth may also in part be owing to its high antioxidant and anti-bacterial capacity.

A 2016 study showed that lavender oil applied topically exhibited a significant hair growth-promoting effect in mice.[17] It increased the number of hair follicles, deepened follicle depth and lowered the quantity of mast cells, indicating a decrease in inflammation. Lavender oil also has antimicrobial properties.

In a 2014 study, a topical treatment of peppermint (*Mentha piperita*) was shown to promote more hair growth in mice than a 3 percent solution of minoxidil.[18] Peppermint increased dermal thickness as well as follicle number, length and depth. It also promoted blood circulation by relaxing vascular smooth muscle which the researchers said may have contributed to an earlier growth phase.

Other good choices of herbs to infuse in oils are nettle, neem, curry leaf, cloves and sage.

Scalp Massage

A regular scalp massage improves circulation by increasing both blood flow towards the hair follicles and lymph flow in the scalp. This, in turn, enhances the supply of nutrients needed for healthy hair growth and assists in removing any toxins. It promotes relaxation, feels good and is a great way to relieve general anxiety and fatigue. For any kind of noticeable results though, it takes long-term daily commitment.

A scalp massage has been shown to increase hair thickness as well as lowering both stress hormones and blood pressure.[19,20] In a 2019 survey daily massage of eleven to twenty minutes for eight months showed hair loss stabilization or reversal in around 75 percent of participants, regardless of age.[21] It can also relieve scalp tension.[22] Tensile forces generated by fibrous tissue underlying the scalp possibly play an important role in the development of MPB.[23,24] When muscle tension is increased, blood supply to the area is reduced. So a regular scalp massage increases blood flow which may reduce the effects of fibrosis. However, as previously noted, a scalp massage only treats the symptoms of fibrosis rather than one of its causes.

A scalp massage can be easily incorporated into your daily routine. You can use your fingers or a simple massage tool like a brush with large rounded wooden bristles. Do not use any tools made from plastic as these may create friction and damage the hair. It's a good idea to cut your fingernails short, so they don't snag at any hairs or scratch the skin and cause unnecessary damage. If you lose some hairs while massaging your head, don't worry about it. They were all probably in the resting phase and were ready to fall out anyway. You are not contributing to your overall loss.

Either sit or lie down in a comfortable position. The fewer distractions the better as you concentrate all your positive energies on the scalp and hair. Start by placing the fingertips of both hands at the hairline, and using a push and pull motion stretch and scrunch the scalp forward and backward. The fingertips remain in place as you feel the scalp move across the skull. The idea is to enhance mobility while increasing blood supply to the whole area. You can stay in the same spot for around twenty seconds or so. Step by step, make your way to the crown and then to the back of your head. Reverse the direction and return to the hairline. Try covering the entire surface of your scalp and not just the areas that are losing hair.

Another technique is to tap the fingertips of both hands up and down on the scalp with a steady rhythm. It is possible to apply a fair amount of pressure but not enough to feel pain or discomfort. This can also be done across the entire scalp. To finish you can use both hands to grasp the hair, if it's long enough. Lightly pull and hold for around five to ten seconds. Don't pull on the length of the hair but just tug near the scalp to gently lift the skin. Release and repeat.

Styling Products

The same general idea applies to styling products as to your choice of shampoo and conditioner: don't use anything that contains harsh chemicals. If you colour your hair, try using organic dyes like henna and indigo powder. Avoid synthetic dyes and bleaches. These contain harsh chemicals which cause scalp irritation and damage hair. Using bleach or man-made colourants involves penetrating the cuticle with chemicals and removing your natural pigment. Herbal colourants, on the other hand, act more like a stain. For more information about naturally dyeing your hair I highly recommend Christine Shahin's book *Natural Hair Coloring*.

There isn't anything terribly wrong with using a brush but it isn't exactly great either. They have a tendency to tear roughly through the hair, putting a lot of physical stress on the cuticle causing breakage and split ends. Instead, try using a wooden wide-toothed comb which is anti-static and doesn't tend to pull or destroy the hair. Your movements too tend to be gentler when using a comb. Wooden combs also prevent the hair from drying out as they help to distribute oil from the scalp to your hair. They just have a much softer feel than plastic or metal, which can catch and snag, as well as damaging the top layer of skin of the scalp. In addition, plastic tends to rip out hair since it causes static. For that same reason, stay away from all plastic hairstyling or massage tools.

Combs though become dirty over time and you don't want to transfer grease or germs back into your hair. However, wood doesn't like water as it can cause the comb to rot or swell and eventually splinter. Instead, you can use oil for cleaning. Dip a clean piece of cloth in any natural oil, then remove dirt or debris from the comb by running the fabric through each tine. You can also scrub the comb gently with an old toothbrush and a weak solution of washing soda (sodium carbonate).

Natural Hair Care

Do not comb hair until it is dry, as damp hair is fragile and tends to break. Your hair is very elastic when wet, so you need to be gentle in detangling it. If you rub your head roughly with a towel, the friction pulls out hair and causes mechanical damage to the cuticles. Allow it to air dry whenever possible or gently pat with a towel. Definitely do not use a blow dryer. This removes not only the surface moisture but also water bound to the hair shafts. The cuticles can then become dry and brittle causing them to crack. Exposing unprotected hair to strong direct sunlight over prolonged periods damages it in a similar way.

Washing with water that is too hot can dehydrate your hair and scalp. This can make hair brittle and more prone to breakage as well as leading to overproduction of sebum. I recommend using warm water and then rinse with cold at the end. Warm water opens the cuticle, so you can easily remove any dirt, product build-up and excess oils. It also makes sure your hair will effectively absorb everything you put on it when adding a conditioner. Rinsing with cold water helps with closing the cuticles so your hair doesn't get damaged too easily after washing. Cold water also improves the blood circulation to your scalp though on the down side it can make your hair look less dense and reduce its volume.

When hair is subjected to prolonged or excessive tension from any source, it can lead to damage. At first hair begins to shed but if the tension persists then it eventually causes hair growth to slow and even stop. Any hairstyle which requires a tight restraint like a ponytail or wearing tightly-fitting caps or hats should be avoided. If you have longer hair then *never* use rubber bands with no fabric coating as this has been shown to destroy the cuticles. Don't wear hats when you have wet hair as this also puts unnecessary stress on the hair shafts.

Choose hats made from unbleached natural fibres such as organic cotton, wool and hemp. Synthetic fibres like polyester, nylon or acrylic are more susceptible to static problems and use various toxic chemicals in their manufacturing. For the same reasons, select a natural fibre (preferably organic and unbleached) for your pillowcase. For some men, sleeping on a cotton pillowcase can cause dryness. If your hair gets matted, tangled or breaks while you sleep: try using a silk pillowcase.

Trim any split ends you may have every six to eight weeks, as they have the tendency to crack and break. A hair cut doesn't affect the overall rate of growth but it does eliminate split ends that may be impeding the growth of individual hairs.

Part 6: Lifestyle Choices

AVOIDING TOXINS

"For the first time in the history of the world, every human being is now subjected to contact with dangerous chemicals, from the moment of conception until death." Rachel Carson

We are surrounded by toxins. They are everywhere in our life and many of them you can't see, feel or smell. Many of these substances didn't exist one hundred and fifty years ago. They are found in our water and food supply, medicines, plastics, personal-care products and cleaning items. We are exposed to small amounts every day, so their effects are insidious. This has become an unfortunate reality of modern life. The majority of us are carrying around some toxic elements stored in our bodies and they most certainly contribute to the issues that cause hair loss. You need a strategy not only to avoid these substances but also to remove them from your body.

It is important to understand where these poisonous chemicals are found, their possible effects and how to avoid them. There is a huge variation in each person's toxin exposure as well as their susceptibility and ability to eliminate them from their body. Once absorbed by our bodily tissues, various toxic compounds tend to remain because they aren't easily broken down and excreted. Diet is the primary source though there are many other causes. Many of the items we take for granted actually contain noxious compounds. Most of us have assumed that products such as plastic are inert or that their negative impact is minimal. Or probably you just haven't given it much thought.

Considering we spend 80 to 90 percent of our lives indoors, where most of our exposure occurs, it is incredibly important to know what products can lead to problems. You have the choice to live, in your own body as well as your home, in either a healthy or unhealthy space. Once you have identified substances that are negatively affecting your health, then you need actively to avoid them. This means not using or buying them and changing a few things around your home and workplace. Initially, this may seem overwhelming, which just goes to show how many are ubiquitous in our lives. For every toxic product you have in your house, there's a non-toxic alternative available. A guide to buying safer products and knowing which one to avoid can be found at: www.lesstoxicguide.ca.

Chlorine, Fluorine and Bromine

Chlorine, fluorine, bromine and iodine are known as halogens and are antagonistic to each other in the body. Increase the level of one or more of them and they tend to replace or remove the others. Iodine is highly beneficial: chlorine, fluorine and bromine are all toxic. These three dangerous halogens have more than likely accumulated in your body through daily routine exposure. It's unrealistic to expect to remove them from all aspects of your life but you can do many things to reduce your exposure, especially in your own home.

•Increase your dietary intake of iodine. This will naturally displace the toxic halogens. Many men in the US and the UK are iodine deficient.

•Avoid drinking unfiltered tap water since it typically contains both chlorine and fluoride. Japan and most of Western Europe have banned fluoridated water though not the US or the UK. Your water supply may also have various xenoestrogens, medications like antibiotics and birth control hormones, as well as heavy metals such as lead. Installing either a reverse osmosis filtration system or some kind of carbon-filtration could eliminate the worst of these, though fluoride is relatively difficult to remove.

The addition of chlorine to drinking water has been found to alter negatively the gut microbiome[1] while high fluoride exposure can cause functional abnormalities of the thyroid.[2] Researchers on this second study concluded that: "*The results…question the validity of the fluoridation of drinking water.*"

•Avoid showering, bathing or swimming in chlorinated water. A shower filter is a great investment. It is not necessarily the chemical itself that causes problems but a wide range of potential by-products that form. Researchers have found that swimming in chlorinated pools may directly lower testosterone levels.[3]

•Sodium fluoride and other chemicals best avoided are added to most toothpaste. Many commercial mouthwashes also contain halogens and other toxic ingredients like triclosan. Your mouth has some of the most absorptive membranes in your body, so some of these chemicals make their way directly into your bloodstream. There are numerous brands of toothpaste available including Dr. Bronner's, Weleda and Nature's Gate that are fluoride-free.

In a 2010 *in vitro* study, exposure to high levels of fluoride compromised hair growth and led to hair loss.[4] The researchers also found the toxicity of fluoride can be reduced by selenium, at least partially via the suppression of oxidative stress. In addition, one review showed that high levels of fluorine were able to: increase calcification of blood vessels; accelerate ageing; reduce testosterone in men; suppress thyroid function and induce oxidative stress.[5] Yet another study found that a low dose of sodium fluoride caused decreased activity of the antioxidant SOD while increasing levels of lipid peroxidation.[6]

•Avoid cooking with non-stick pans as these can significantly increase the fluoride content of food (Teflon contains perfluorinated compounds or PFCs). Switch to ceramic, stainless steel, cast iron or those with a coating that are certified to contain no fluoride. PFCs are also found in grease-resistant packaging such as wrappers for burgers and sandwiches, pizza boxes and popcorn bags. Many brands of dental floss are coated with Teflon and PFCs can also be found in shaving cream. Watch out for ingredients containing the word 'fluoro' or 'perfluoro.' Animal studies with PFCs have been linked to liver toxicity, lower testosterone levels and decreased thyroid hormones.[7]

•Some soda drinks, especially citrus flavour, contain bromine (brominated vegetable oil or BVO) such as Mountain Dew, Gatorade and Squirt. Avoid all of them. BVO is banned in the UK and the European Union as it's linked to thyroid issues and reproductive interference. Bromine may also be added to commercial baked goods as an anti-caking or bleaching agent, as well as a fumigant to stored grains.

•Brominated flame retardants can be found in mattresses, carpets, car seats and various textiles. These chemicals have been shown to block testosterone production,[8] alter thyroid hormones and are associated with increased risk of metabolic syndrome.[9] Research any products especially furniture and mattresses that you buy.

•Plenty of household cleaners don't contain chlorine and other toxic substances. Companies such as Method, Seventh Generation, Ecover and Ecos make non-toxic cleaning products.

•Be aware that many common drugs contain fluorine and bromine, including antacids, antibiotics and antihistamines. Many multi-mineral pills also have fluorides added.

Synthetic Xenoestrogens

This group of man-made chemicals is a type of endocrine disruptor that mimics the effects of the hormone oestrogen. You absorb them by ingestion, inhalation or direct skin contact. Synthetic xenoestrogens entering the skin go directly to the tissues of the body without passing through the liver for detoxification: so they can potentially be far more potent than those consumed orally. They are then stored in your fat cells. Researchers found that synthetic xenoestrogens such as BPA and parabens are able to act together to produce a cumulative effect when combined.[10] They tested mixtures of xenoestrogens and found they produced significant results even when each component was combined at concentrations below a level that had no observed effect. They concluded that: *"Our results highlight the limitations of the traditional focus on the effects of single agents. Hazard assessments that ignore the possibility of joint action of oestrogenic chemicals will almost certainly lead to significant underestimations of risk."*

Limit your contact to as many of these chemicals as possible. Simple steps can make a significant difference. The problem is we are exposing our bodies to these foreign oestrogens all the time: every day of the year and constantly activating our oestrogen receptors unnecessarily.

Food and Water: Another reason to avoid unfiltered tap water is the presence of pharmaceuticals used to treat millions of farm animals against illness and infections. Atrazine, arsenic and perchlorate are three endocrine disruptors present in many water supplies. Install a filter for all drinking, cooking and showering.

•Buy hormone-free animal products. This is important to avoid the various hormones, chemicals and steroids that are fed to factory-farmed animals such as zeranol, an anabolic growth promoter and a known synthetic xenoestrogen.

•Buy organic fruit and vegetables if available. Wash or peel non-organic fruits and vegetables. Many pesticides and other biocides are xenoestrogens as well as containing chlorine and bromine. Organic food contains fewer xenoestrogens and other chemicals, both sprayed on the surface of the produce and absorbed from the soil.

•Avoid foods with the additives propyl gallate (E310), BHA (E320) and BHT (E321): all synthetic xenoestrogens. These preservatives can be found in many products including vegetable oil, butter and various processed foods that contain fats and oils.

•Avoid fast and processed food. Apart from the low quality frying oils, another problem is a group of chemicals called phthalates. They're used to make plastics soft and flexible, and are found in many products ranging from soda bottles to plastic bags (also in personal-care products, laundry detergents and air fresheners). Food can be a major source of exposure as packaging materials and equipment contains phthalates, and these chemicals leach into whatever they are in contact with. Any food highly processed, packaged and handled may be a significant source. Fast food, processed meats (especially poultry), fats and dairy products are those most likely to be contaminated.[11,12]

176 men were tested over a period of two years, and researchers found that exposure to phthalates led to a significant decrease in testosterone levels.[13]

Plastic and Cans: The chemical BPA (bisphenol-A) is often found in various plastic containers and is a known synthetic xenoestrogen. For most people, ingestion of contaminated food contributes to more than 90 percent of exposure.

Researchers looking at various plastics concluded that: "*Almost all commercially available plastic products we sampled— independent of the type of resin, product, or retail source—leached chemicals having reliably detectable EA* [estrogenic activity], *including those advertised as BPA free. In some cases, BPA-free products released chemicals having more EA than did BPA-containing products.*"[14]

In one review it was stated that: "*In the United States, exposure to BPA is widespread, exceeding 90 percent in the general population. Dermal absorption, inhalation, and ingestion from contaminated food and water are the major routes of exposure. As an endocrine disruptor that mimics estrogen and thyroid hormone, BPA also acts as a metabolic and immune disruptor. Thus, the adverse health effects of BPA are extensive, and higher levels of BPA exposure correlate with increased risk of cardiovascular disease, obesity, diabetes, immune disorders, and a host of reproductive dysfunctions.*"[15]

Another review revealed that male workers exposed to BPA are at a greater risk of dysfunction across *all* domains of sexual function.[16] It also showed that although BPA is considered a weak oestrogen, it can promote oestrogen-like effects similar to or stronger than oestradiol (the most powerful natural oestrogen).

Some people are buying 'BPA-free' products believing this label must equate to something that is either good or at least non-toxic. Unfortunately, this is not true. Manufacturers have been replacing BPA with bisphenol analogs (such as BPS or BPZ) and they seem to have similar endocrine disruption properties.

To avoid exposure to xenoestrogens such as BPA and phthalates in your food you can try some of these recommendations:

•Use stainless steel or glass water bottles. Try eliminating all dietary liquids stored in plastics, especially oils. Buy food in glass jars. The bottoms of most plastic containers have a triangle with a number inside it. The general rule is to choose recyclable plastic #1, #2, #4 or #5. Avoid #3 (PVC), #6 (polystyrene) and #7 (BPA or BPS). Also avoid those marked with 'PC' for polycarbonate. Some plastics may contain up to 40 percent phthalates.

•Never microwave or heat plastic with food inside. It is worth reducing your exposure to food in contact with plastic, particularly if it is hot, liquid or acidic.

•Use glass containers at home for storage. With each use and wash, disposable plastic breaks down, increasing the potential for chemicals to leach into your food and drink.

•Stop using plastic wrap and remove any on products that you buy. Researchers measured over 900 food contact materials with their potential to bind to the oestrogen receptor and cause adverse effects.[17] They found seven chemicals including BPA had a very strong affinity to bind to the oestrogen receptor even at extremely low concentrations and concluded that: *"These substances represent a real threat to the health of the population."*

•Use all glass and/or stainless steel kitchen appliances such as coffee makers and kettles. Avoid plastic or silicone utensils.

•Take away cups are generally fused with polyethylene (a synthetic xenoestrogen) to make it waterproof. BPA is also found in disposable coffee lids.

•Try avoiding all products that contain PVC (polyvinyl chloride). PVC contains phthalates, dioxins and furans: all potent xenoestrogens. Toxic metals are also commonly used in the manufacture of this plastic. PVC is found in many everyday products such as wrapping film for food, imitation leather, raincoats, furniture and older water pipes. In one study five PVC shower curtains were tested and all were found to contain volatile organic compounds (VOCs), phthalates and one or more of the heavy metals: lead, cadmium, mercury and chromium.[18] Cotton, linen or hemp shower curtains can be used instead. Hemp is a strong natural fibre that requires considerably fewer pesticides during its production compared with other traditional crops.

•Stop eating food out of cans as the sealant used for the liner is almost always made from synthetic xenoestrogens. For the same reason, most commercial juice cartons should be avoided. Aluminium cans for sodas are lined with BPA.

Personal-Care Products: It's not enough just to replace your shampoo and conditioner as the majority of deodorants, sunscreen, aftershave, soap, toothpaste, mouthwash and shaving cream all contain synthetic xenoestrogens. Try to purchase and store all your personal-care products in glass containers.

•The majority of deodorants have harmful ingredients including parabens (synthetic xenoestrogens) and aluminium compounds (toxic and xenoestrogenic). Most deodorants like Axe, Old Spice and Right Guard should all be avoided. There are many natural brands available such as Nature's Gate and For Pit's Sake.

•Common sunscreen ingredients oxybenzone, 4-MBC, benzophenones and PABA are all xenoestrogens. If your sunscreen contains any of these chemicals then use another brand. Most also have a base made of some PUFA. One review concluded that: *"Numerous studies raised concerns about the association between exposure to substances commonly found in sunscreens and endocrine and developmental impairments."*[19] There are many brands available without these toxic chemicals like those made by Aubrey Organics and Babo Botanicals. The best protection against unwanted ultraviolet light is a good tan, a hat or other protective clothing.

•If your aftershave, soap or shaving cream contains the ingredient fragrance (parfum), then stop using it. They probably contain parabens and phthalates. Natural shaving creams are available from companies such as Avalon Organics and Green People.

•Research ingredients in your pharmaceuticals as these can also contain synthetic xenoestrogens.

Household and Gardening Products: Indoor air is typically two to five times more polluted than outdoor air. Ventilate your house frequently as toxins can come from carpets, rugs and furniture. Clean, dust and vacuum your house regularly. Try choosing household and laundry alternatives, as well as any gardening products, that are less toxic than standard.

•Do not use plug-in air fresheners, scented sprays or candles as they probably contain parabens and phthalates (listed as fragrances or parfum).

•Try avoiding regular laundry and dishwashing detergents, household cleaners and dryer sheets which can all contain artificial fragrances (xenoestrogens). One common ingredient found in detergent that should definitely be avoided is nonylphenol (highly xenoestrogenic): its use has been restricted in the European Union but not the US. There are plenty of natural brands of cleaning products like Seventh Generation and Ecover. Don't trust it just because it says 'green' or 'natural' on the label. Some of the most useful non-toxic cleaning products are baking soda, castile soap, vinegar and lemon juice.

•It is important to remove all moulds from your home, especially your bedroom and bathroom, no matter what type it is. This will reduce your exposure to mycotoxins. Ventilate your bathroom, laundry and cooking areas and fix any leaks or water damage you have around the house. Clean areas that have mould growing or replace items such as carpets and shower curtains.

•If you have a garden, stop using all conventional pesticides and chemicals. Pesticides are also found in mothballs, bug sprays and flea repellent. These products all contain xenoestrogens.

•Plants are living filters that help to reduce indoor air pollution. Whether you are aware of it or not, there are many potentially harmful gases and other contaminants inside your home. These include formaldehyde, VOCs and airborne biological pollutants such as pollen and moulds, some of which are xenoestrogens. NASA scientists in the late '80s and early '90s found that certain plants were very effective at absorbing these toxins. English ivy, Boston ferns, lady palm, garden mum, spider plant, peace lily, bamboo palm, chrysanthemums and aloe vera are some of the plants best at removing these contaminants. Plants absorb some of the particulates from the air at the same time as they take in carbon dioxide. The microorganisms present in the soil are also responsible for much of the cleaning effect. Beyond air quality, plants just make you feel better.

Toxic Heavy Metals

They exist all around us; hidden in our water and food, around our house and even in the air we breathe. Some of them are only dangerous in large quantities, whilst trace amounts of others may be detrimental. Acute exposure may come from the workplace if you work with metals, plastics or ceramics. Some professions with extremely high exposure include battery makers, jewellers, solderers, roofers, printers, dentists and gasoline attendants. For most people contact happens slowly over time, usually a matter of years.

We have both toxic and nutrient metals in our body. Toxic metals should not be there and serve no biological function, whereas nutrient metals such as zinc are fundamental to health. If you're deficient in an essential mineral, your body will use a toxic heavy metal in its place. Sometimes you can drive out an unwanted metal from the body by simply increasing a nutrient metal that is low. Certain heavy metals in excess can activate the oestrogen receptor and these are sometimes referred to as metallooestrogens. These include mercury, lead, cadmium and arsenic.[20]

Mercury: Exposure occurs via inhalation, skin absorption or ingestion. Common sources are air pollution, amalgam 'silver' dental fillings (typically around 55 percent mercury), vaccines containing thimerosal as well as dietary exposure, most commonly via contaminated seafood. It can also be present in HFCS.

Try having your amalgam fillings replaced with a composite material that is BPA-free. Many dentists specialize in this procedure. In one review researchers stated that: *"Dental amalgam is by far the main source of human total mercury body burden. This is proven by autopsy studies which found 2-12 times more mercury in body tissues of individuals with dental amalgam."*[21] They also go on to say that amalgams reduce glutathione levels, aggravate a deficiency of selenium and significantly increase oxidative stress. These issues are directly correlated with the numbers of fillings.

Lead: Exposure to this metal is known to cause an accumulation in male reproductive organs and induce infertility. Those with the highest amounts in their bodies have been shown to produce more cortisol in response to routine stressors.[22] Common sources of toxic exposure include lead-based paints, contaminated water, seafood, air pollution, gasoline products, hair dye and PVC.

Cadmium: This metal is present in many foods, with the heaviest contamination found in shellfish, liver and kidney meats. Conventional crops also contain significantly higher concentrations than organic. Cadmium is found in PVC and other plastics, as well as contaminated air and tobacco smoke (including e-cigarettes). This toxic metal is more easily absorbed if you are deficient in zinc, selenium, calcium or iron. Several dietary recommendations have been found to help with cadmium and lead toxicity: these include eating more tomatoes, berries, onions, garlic and grapes.[23]

In a 2015 study, researchers suggested that elevated levels of cadmium and lead may be a hidden cause of hair loss.[24] These toxic metals cause oxidative damage and reduce levels of various antioxidants including glutathione. Furthermore, cadmium has been shown to displace testosterone from its receptors (effectively reducing overall levels) and induce tissue injury through increased lipid peroxidation.[25] Effective antioxidant therapies suggested in the study included dietary zinc, selenium and the vitamins A, C and E, which may antagonize these negative effects.

Arsenic: Exposure of this metalloid occurs mostly in the workplace but can come from various sources. These include treated wood, paint, water, air pollution as well as contaminated seafood, poultry, pork, flour, corn, rice and tofu. Many chickens and pigs raised in the US are given feed that contains a form of arsenic. When a person absorbs excessive amounts, it is deposited in the hair, nails and skin. Foods high in selenium such as Brazil nuts are a potential countermeasure against accumulation and toxicity induced by both arsenic and cadmium.[26]

Whilst there is no way to avoid exposure to heavy metals altogether, it can be significantly reduced by limiting consumption of fish and seafood; installing a water purification system; removing any amalgam fillings; removing all PVC products from your home; you are ensuring getting enough nutrient metals such as zinc, magnesium and selenium in your diet; increasing your intake of antioxidants such as glutathione and vitamins A, C and E; eating more organic food and stopping smoking. Keep in mind that removing the sources of exposure is the single most important principle.

If you are concerned about an acute exposure to heavy metals, then blood, urine and hair are all reasonable places to look for signs of toxicity. If your levels are high, you can consider chelation therapy under a doctor's supervision. Alternatively, fasting will safely remove these toxins.

Detoxification and Fasting
"The best of all medicines is resting and fasting." Benjamin Franklin

Detoxification is when your body rids itself of unwanted chemicals stored in the cells and tissues and puts them back into the blood for elimination. The term is also applied to describe a treatment intended to improve or assist this process by using specific foods, supplements and herbs. Fasting increases antioxidant activity[27] and is nature's way of detoxing the body.

In my experience, the greatest benefit is to help you change to a long-term, healthier way of eating and living. It's a good time to reflect on the conscious relationship you have with your body. Fasting is somewhat pointless if you immediately return to all your bad habits. However, toxins don't accumulate in only a week: therefore, they aren't going to disappear after one short fast either. You need to build healthy and sustainable habits that help you deal with the toxic burden we encounter every single day. Fasting is only one of those tools.

Researchers studied the fat from twenty people and found nineteen different substances that were oestrogenic (or likely to be oestrogenic) including BPA, benzophenones, triclosan and parabens in all twenty subjects.[28] These results suggest that fat (adipose) tissue is an important repository for xenoestrogens. We all have some toxins stored inside us and these can include toxic heavy metals, various synthetic xenoestrogens, moulds and VOCs such as formaldehyde. These stored toxins will be released as you are fasting.

Before starting a juice fast, it is important to ensure you have a healthy microbiome and are not nutrient deficient. Sufficient amounts of magnesium, selenium, sulphur, vitamin B_9 (folate), vitamin B_{12} and the antioxidant glutathione are all necessary to remove toxins from the body. DO NOT attempt a juice fast if your health is compromised. If you are heavily toxic and want to fast, then please seek professional supervision. Although that sounds paradoxical, you need a certain level of health otherwise released toxins cannot be excreted from your body.

There are many different ways to fast and I recommend a juice fast. This involves consuming nothing but fresh vegetable juices, herbal teas, fibre and water for a predetermined length of time. It is recommended to fast for three to ten days, a few times a year. Ten days may seem like a very long time to go without food, though fasting is not as uncomfortable as many would think. Some important components of a successful juice fast include:

1) Juice: You should be drinking at least two vegetable juices a day. There are several foods that have been shown to help with detoxification. These include alliums (onion, shallots, garlic, scallions [spring onions], leek and chives), cruciferous vegetables (cauliflower, cabbage, broccoli, Brussels sprouts, garden cress, kale, spring greens, rocket, radish, watercress and bok choy), asparagus, lemon, lime, bean sprouts, beetroot and ginger root.[29,30,31] You can also add cucumber to make these juices more palatable.

On the other hand there are a few foods that have been shown to block detoxification. Surprisingly these include carrot, celery, parsley and coriander.[32]

2) Sauna and Exercise: Gentle exercise and sauna are extremely important on a fast. Exercise mobilizes toxins while both exercise and sauna help to excrete them. The body is able to sweat out toxic materials including the heavy metals arsenic, cadmium, lead and mercury; synthetic xenoestrogens and mycotoxins. Many cultures have used saunas for cleansing, relaxing and rejuvenating purposes and there is considerable evidence to show how beneficial they are

for your health.[33,34,35,36]

3) Herbal Tea: These can be enjoyed throughout the day as you fast. St. John's wort, chamomile, chicory root, dandelion root, burdock root, rooibos and honeybush tea have all been shown to be beneficial to detoxification pathways.[29,37,38]

4) Binding Agents and Fibre: While fasting you're primarily burning fat as fuel and this releases the toxins stored within the fat cells and other tissues. To avoid these toxins being reabsorbed, it's important to help your body to remove them completely. As well as drinking herbal tea there are various products that can help you with this process.

a) Activated carbon (charcoal) binds to organic toxins such as mycotoxins, so they can be excreted from the body.[39] Choose a brand made from coconut shells or other natural sources without any additives or fillers. Take around five to ten grams at least one hour before drinking any juices, no less than once per day. It's important to drink plenty of water when using activated charcoal.

b) Soluble and insoluble fibre work to clean the digestive tract of waste and toxins and help remove them from the body. Psyllium is produced from the seeds and husks of the plant. The husk is approximately 70 percent soluble fibre while the seeds are almost entirely insoluble fibre. Most psyllium supplements only have the husks, so find one that also contains the seeds. Psyllium can be consumed in doses of five to ten grams with your juices, at least once per day.

c) Bentonite clay helps to remove various toxins from the body such as mould toxins, pesticides, lead and cadmium.[40] Mix around a half to a full teaspoon with water and drink immediately. Consume on an empty stomach at least one hour before a juice or taking another supplement. This can be taken up to three times daily. Remember to drink lots of water when using clay.

Chlorella, spirulina and blue-green algae are not particularly effective at binding to toxins, but can be taken for their nutritional value. However, do not take any 'detox' supplements especially anything that is concentrated beyond what is found in nature.

5) Stay hydrated: As well as fresh juice and tea, it is advisable to drink plenty of filtered water. Staying hydrated is extremely important when on a juice cleanse. Water will help to not only flush toxins from your system, but also to keep sensations of hunger at bay.

Before the fast: Decide how many days you will be fasting. You will need large quantities of fresh vegetables, preferably organic and a good quality juicer. If you do not have a water filter at home, stock up on some spring water. Timing is important when it comes to fasting. You will need to ensure there are no high-energy activities planned for the period. Allow yourself time to rest and know it's easier to do when the weather is warmer.

During the fast: Whenever you feel hungry or thirsty, drink a juice, water or a herbal tea. Gentle movement is vital during cleansing to assist the lymphatic system expel toxins. Thirty to forty-five minutes a day of low-impact movement such as walking, stretching or yoga is recommended. Avoid any intense workouts. Getting a full body massage will also stimulate the body to release toxins. Headaches, fatigue, aches, irritability, body odour and general malaise are common for as many as four or five days into the fast as your body cleans itself out. On the other hand, you might experience positive sensations such as exuberance, deep and restoring sleep, a feeling of lightness and sharpened senses.

After the fast: It's important to break your fast correctly by consuming, for example, some fruit on the first morning. Ease your body out slowly by eating lightly for a few days. The longer the fasting period, the gentler you must be. The most important thing to remember is not to eat too much as there is a natural tendency to overeat as soon as the fast is over.

Ways to Reduce Stress

"Stress can wreak havoc with your metabolism, raise your blood pressure, burst your white blood cells, make you flatulent, ruin your sex life, and if that's not enough, possibly damage your brain."
Robert M. Sapolsky, Why Zebras Don't Get Ulcers

The common misconception with stress is that it is only an emotional problem, often disguised as anxiety, worry or depression. However, the reality is that any stimulus, no matter whether chemical, emotional or physical, that is perceived by the body as challenging, threatening or demanding can be labelled as a stressor. A wide range of chemicals and hormones modulate the body's response to stress, and some of these can negatively alter hair growth. Having said that, we are all individuals and no two people respond exactly the same to any given stressor.

Chemical stress is caused by an imbalance in the body. The main reasons are either internal such as diet, smoking, alcohol and drugs, or external including pollution and exposure to toxic chemicals. Emotional stress happens when we judge any event negatively. Work, family, relationships and city life can all be significant sources. Physical stress is not usually something drastic or obvious like a wound but normally it's more subtle, such as sitting down for long periods of time or repetitive lifting and bending. Everyday activities involve postures that create indistinct stress, strain and injury. Since most of us are using computers or sitting for longer periods of time, we are potentially maintaining stressful postures and body positions. Most of us are also neither exercising nor moving enough.

In a 2003 study the researchers showed for the first time that emotional stress negatively alters the hair cycle in mice by reducing the growth stage.[41] They also showed inflammation was present in the stressed mice indicated by excessive mast cell activation and other markers.

A 2019 study examined 13,391 employed men.[42] It was found that men who worked more than fifty-two hours a week lost their hair at twice the speed of those spending less than forty hours at work. The lead researcher stated: *"The results of this study demonstrate that long working hours is significantly associated with the increased development of alopecia in male workers. A lot of studies have revealed the mechanism of alopecia development by stress.*" These results demonstrate that hair loss can be mediated by job-related stress and the strength of association increases linearly as work time gets longer.

Stress is meant to protect you from immediate physical danger and much of this physiological response was laid down through thousands of years of evolution. However, the body does not seem to recognise the social transformation of humans. It assesses all situations as though 'fight or flight' stance has to be maintained, even with stresses associated with work in an office. Stress is unavoidable but just because it is common in our modern life, that does not make it natural. While cortisol is a critical and helpful part of the stress response, it's important that the body returns to a neutral mode after a stressful event. Unfortunately in our current culture, the stress response is activated so often that the body doesn't always have a chance to return to normal, resulting in a state of chronic stress. We've become so obsessed with always being *on* that we've lost the ability to turn ourselves *off.*

As we have already seen in part 2, stress is an enemy of a balanced hormonal system. It raises cortisol, oestrogen and prolactin while decreasing thyroid and androgen levels. Certain herbs, exercise, healthy eating habits, meditation, changing sleep patterns and cultivating positive relationships can all help to reduce chronic stress and stress-related inflammation. This means developing new habits which takes time, effort and persistence. It may not always be possible to make our lives or the world around us less stressful but you can do a lot to control it. Any regime to help hair loss must include ways to decrease all forms of stress: chemical, emotional and physical.

•Physical exercise is one of the best ways to remove excessive stress hormones and restore your body and mind to a calmer, more relaxed state. Exercise and the self-discipline it involves help you respond effectively to any problems and make you feel stronger and confident in the face of stress. It can also give you more energy to get things done. Regular physical activity will also improve the quality of your sleep and remove toxins from your body.

Engaging in sedentary activities to deal with stress is quite common. Watching TV or surfing the internet may seem great ways to zone out after a hard day but both stimulate your nervous system and reduce your ability to relax. Instead try engaging in a suitable exercise activity you naturally enjoy. It's easy to find excuses, especially when you are stressed or busy. Good intentions aren't enough. You have to take specific steps to translate your desires into action and deal with the inevitable obstacles.

•Take a walk in nature or somewhere outdoors. Exposure to natural light has been shown to decrease stress levels.[43]

•Yoga and meditation are great methods to reduce stress and change the way you react to a difficult situation.[44,45] Regular practices can improve your sleep and increase antioxidant levels.[46] Yoga can also help your digestion, relieve tension, improve your posture and increase blood flow and circulation to your scalp, especially after inverted postures (see appendix C). Meditation isn't difficult to learn and do but requires commitment, patience and practice. You can perform each morning or in the evening just before bed. Meditation on a regular basis lowers levels of both cortisol and adrenaline (epinephrine). The best way to learn yoga and meditation is to take a class with an experienced teacher.

•Get a massage. Much of our psychological anxiety and stress is held in our physical body. Manipulation of the muscles can be extremely helpful in removing tension and training the body to release stress as it builds. Massage also significantly decreases cortisol levels.[47] There are many different types, from gentle to deep tissue work. As with most therapies, you need to decide which form works best.

•Adaptogenic herbs allow our body to handle a stressful situation in a more resourceful manner. It is believed they work by increasing the ability of cells to manufacture and use fuel more efficiently. Some recommended adaptogens are ashwagandha, He shou wu, mucuna pruriens and eleuthero. Other herbs that reduce stress and help you to relax include kava-kava, rhodiola rosea, *Bacopa monnieri* (Brahmi) and valerian root. You can drink three to four cups of tea a day or take as a tincture.

•Choosing healthy foods can positively impact your mood, relieve tension, stabilize blood sugar and reduce stress levels. Good choices include those rich in vitamin B_9 (folate) like dark leafy greens, asparagus and avocado, as well as foods high in vitamin C such as fresh fruit. Resilience to environmental stress appears to be heavily influenced by the composition of your microbiome.[48] Therefore, it's best to avoid refined grains, chemical preservatives, sugar substitutes and other unnatural substances. Paradoxically, when dealing with stress, the body frequently craves precisely the foods that will exacerbate the condition. Consuming unhealthy foods in response to stress or as a way to calm down is very common. It can also happen because you lack time and energy. Eating your meals on a regular schedule and planning them in advance can prevent this problem.

•Common food allergens such as gluten, casein in dairy products, soy, peanuts, corn and chicken eggs have been shown to trigger anxiety, which can stimulate surges in both cortisol and insulin.[49] Check to see if you have any food allergies and avoid products you are sensitive to.

•Avoid, or at least reduce, your consumption of nicotine, excess caffeine and alcohol. Both caffeine and nicotine are stimulants and so will increase your level of stress rather than reduce it. It is common for men to turn to alcohol as a means of dealing with stress. So while alcohol may help deal with the problem in the short-term, in the long run it can contribute to overall levels.

•Try resolving any emotional or financial issues that are worrying you. Stress can be triggered by a problem that may on the surface seem impossible to solve. Learning how to find solutions to your problems will help you feel more in control.

•Make sure you get enough sleep. A lack of sleep is one of the biggest contributors to high cortisol levels. Unfortunately, stress can affect your ability to fall and stay asleep.

How to get a Good Night's Sleep

This is the body's time to detoxify, regenerate and repair your immune and hormonal systems. Sleep increases both testosterone and active thyroid hormone while decreasing cortisol, insulin, prolactin, oestrogen and inflammation.[50] Getting regular quality sleep should be a priority. However, changing our sleep patterns is not something we can do overnight.

The *US Centers for Disease Control and Prevention* reported in 2012 that 30 percent of American adults are sleeping six or fewer hours a night. According to the UK's *Office for National Statistics* survey from 2016, 23 percent of UK adults manage no more than five hours a night. To put things in perspective, in 1910, most people slept around nine hours a night. The right amount though is entirely personal.

Ten healthy young men who underwent a week of sleep deprivation to five hours per night, saw their daytime testosterone decrease by 10 to 15 percent.[51] This lowered testosterone was caused by raised cortisol levels. In other study 531 healthy men aged between twenty-nine and seventy-two were tested.[52] Those who slept four hours per night had 60 percent less testosterone than those sleeping for eight hours. The researchers concluded that sleep duration, independent of age, exercise and body fat was positively associated with testosterone.

A good book about improving your sleep is Shawn Stevenson's *Sleep Smarter: 21 Essential Strategies to Sleep Your Way to a Better Body, Better Health, and Bigger Success*. The reasons we aren't getting enough sleep vary depending upon our lives and circumstances. Even so, there are proven ways to ensure a good night's rest for most people:

•Cycles of light and darkness appear to have a dramatic effect on hair growth. Sleep in complete darkness or as close to it as possible. Use blackout curtains if necessary and an alarm clock that does not glow in the dark. If you go to the bathroom during the night, keep the lights off. Even the tiniest bit of light can disrupt production of the sleep-inducing hormone melatonin. This hormone is secreted only in conditions of darkness and has been shown to: interfere with oestrogen-signalling pathways and function as an anti-oestrogen,[53] improve thyroid function and insulin sensitivity, as well as act as a powerful antioxidant.[54] In addition, it has been found to inhibit action of the toxic metal cadmium.[55]

•Two hours of evening use of a device that emits blue light has been shown to suppress melatonin production by more than 20 percent.[56] New artificial lights such as LED and CFL amplify blue light beyond anything we have evolved to handle. Replace the bulbs in your bedroom with blue-blocking bulbs and avoid all electronics with screens close to your bedtime.

•Reduce electromagnetic fields around where you sleep by moving alarm clocks and other electrical devices such as smartphones and computers away from the bed. Better still: avoid all electronic devices in your bedroom. Switch off your Wi-Fi at night as well. Electric and magnetic fields (invisible forces that surround any electrical device) have been shown to interrupt sleep cycles.

•You sleep better if the temperature in your bedroom is kept on the cool side: so try sleeping with the window open or a fan, as your body temperature drops during the night.

•Try to get up each morning and go to bed every night at roughly the same time. Establishing regular sleeping hours can help you stabilize your internal clocks.

•Most people report it's easier to fall asleep if they have time to wind down into a less active state. Avoid stimulating activities before bed such as watching TV, using the computer, working or exercising. Give yourself adequate time to disengage from mental and physical activity before trying to sleep. Don't work in bed. Keep an uncluttered and peaceful bedroom.

•Avoid eating at least three hours before bed. If there is food still in your stomach, sleep may be disrupted, even if you don't wake up. It may also stop you falling asleep.

•Lose some weight. Being overweight however is a double-edged sword. Not only does an unhealthy weight contribute to sleep problems but also sleep issues can lead to weight gain.

•Willibald Nagler, MD, former chief physiatrist at The New York Hospital-Weill Cornell Medical Center, believed that: *"99.9 percent of the population would sleep better on a firm mattress than a soft one. This holds true for back pain sufferers especially."*

•Sleep naked. Choose bedding made of organic and unbleached cotton or other natural fibres. Wash your bedding regularly in non-toxic detergent to reduce dust mites and other allergens.

•Various herbs have been used through the centuries to treat insomnia. Some good choices are ashwagandha, chamomile, kava-kava, Brahmi, skullcap and valerian root.

•Reduce your consumption of caffeinated drinks, nicotine and alcohol. It can take as long as six to eight hours for the effects of caffeine to wear off completely. Remember it is hidden in many products such as soda.

•Some common prescription and over-the-counter medicines contain caffeine including decongestants, steroids and pain relievers. Avoid sleeping pills unless necessary as they are completely detrimental to your health.

•Spend at least fifteen minutes every day outside in the sun. Daylight is one of the keys to regulating sleep patterns. Sleep troubles are disproportionately more common among those who spend a lot of their time indoors. The body clock is most responsive to sunlight in the early morning.

Exercise and Smoking

Physical exercise is a critical part of healthy living. It stimulates circulation, promotes better sleep, develops muscular tone, decreases body fat, benefits the microbiome[57] and improves posture, as well as self-esteem and body image. Exercise is also one of the best and most natural ways of getting our mental and physical reactions to stress back into balance. Hormonal gains include decreased cortisol, inflammation, insulin, aromatase and oestrogen, as well as increased androgens and thyroid hormone. To optimize your hormonal balance, you need to exercise on a regular basis. Find a suitable exercise activity that you naturally enjoy. Exercise and sweating also both help to remove toxins from your body.

One 2017 study showed that moderate-to-high intensity exercise can reduce hair loss by activating antioxidant defence mechanisms to lower oxidative stress.[58]

However, both high-intensity and prolonged exercise increase prolactin and cortisol, which can remain elevated for hours following a workout. If you exercise excessively, your body is subjected to a state of chronic stress and increased oxidative stress.[59,60] You should work out hard, but feel great and full of energy afterwards. If you are tired or irritable, you are probably training too much. As a general rule, more than an hour on a daily basis is too much. The key is quality of exercise, not quantity.

Smoking is significantly associated with hair loss[61] and smokers are far more likely to go prematurely grey. The carbon monoxide that you inhale prevents the blood from transporting oxygen and key nutrients to hair follicles while the nicotine narrows the blood vessels, further inhibiting growth. Cadmium, a major constituent of tobacco smoke (including e-cigarettes), is toxic and displaces zinc in the body.[62] Other dangerous ingredients in tobacco smoke include acetone, arsenic, benzene and formaldehyde. Smoking also increases the production of the pro-oxidant ROS and levels of oxidative stress in the scalp.[63]

Positive Thinking and Positive Action

"Man often becomes what he believes himself to be. If I keep on saying to myself that I cannot do a certain thing, it is possible that I may end by really becoming incapable of doing it. On the contrary, if I have the belief that I can do it, I shall surely acquire the capacity to do it even if I may not have it at the beginning." Ghandi

Ask yourself every day: what is it that I can do to make my hair healthier? Do not expect anybody else to do it for you. Empower yourself with positive action and thought. Every time you lose a hair, affirm that a new and healthy one will grow in its place. This will help you worry less and care better for your hair. Whenever you look in the mirror, send it love and refrain from thinking or saying anything harsh, even if tempted to do so. Try planting the idea of beautiful healthy hair in the fertile ground of your open mind.

Hair Loss Drugs

"It's a real irony. Men took finasteride to stop or prevent hair loss and sometimes to improve their dating lives. And it actually ended up destroying their sexuality and self-esteem." Dr Irwig, Endocrinologist

Minoxidil and finasteride are the two main drugs with full MHRA (UK) and FDA (US) approval and are recommended by doctors around the world. Even so, both drugs tend only to grow hair on the top and sides of the head: they do not generally produce any at the hairline.

Rogaine (or Regaine) is the brand name for minoxidil. Although this drug has been scientifically proven to have some positive result on hair loss, it has also been shown to have side effects, including: inflammation of hair follicles; a dry, flaky, itchy scalp; spots (acne) developing on the scalp; a burning sensation in the scalp; breast tenderness; decrease in libido; light-headedness; water retention; an *increase* in hair loss; rapid weight gain; vomiting; headaches; fainting; rapid heartbeat or heart palpitations; chest pain (angina); and breathing problems. Children and pregnant women are advised to avoid touching this drug. Some of the ingredients in Rogaine are banned in certain countries because they are considered carcinogenic and tumour-promoting.

Minoxidil is effective in about 30 to 35 percent of men who use the drug. It often takes months of treatment before you know whether it works, or if it's been a complete waste of your time, effort and money. It's also a life-long commitment. You need to use every day for the rest of your life and if you stop, then any hair that has grown back will fall out.

Finasteride, sold under the brand names Proscar and Propecia among others, is another approved medication used for the treatment of MPB. Its effectiveness became known when men taking it for prostate issues grew new hair. You also need to keep taking this drug for life as all new hair will fall out once you stop. Although quite effective for restoring hair growth in many men, there are a number of side effects that include: erectile dysfunction; impotence; testicular pain; complete loss of sexual appetite; clinical depression; prostate cancer; decreased sperm count and quality; breast cancer; and possibly kidney damage.[64] A few men have found that the sexual side effects do not go away once the drug is stopped.

Children and pregnant women are also advised to avoid touching this drug. Dutasteride (sold under the brand name Avodart) has similar side effects.

There is an excellent online article from 2016 written by Lisa Marshall that gives more information about these drugs. It can be found on the website Tonic, entitled *The Medical Mystery Behind America's Best-Selling Hair-loss Drug* (*tonic.vice.com*). Several scientific studies have also been done on these drugs:

In a 2003 study, researchers followed 3,040 men ranging in age from forty-five to seventy-eight, all of whom suffered from prostate enlargement, another condition finasteride is approved to treat.[65] In the study's first year, 15 percent of the men on the drug suffered new sexual side effects, compared with only 7 percent of the men on placebos. The lead researcher had this to say: "*There were real, ill effects from the drug. In some men, finasteride caused erectile dysfunction; in others it decreased ejaculate volume; and in others it reduced libido.*"

A 2014 study on drugs like finasteride came to this conclusion: "*...a substantial body of evidence exists which points to serious and potentially ill-health effects of 5α-RIs' therapy. These include loss or reduced libido, erectile dysfunction, orgasmic and ejaculatory dysfunction, development of high grade PCa tumors, potential negative cardiovascular events, and depression. The side effects are potentially harmful in some individuals and in young men may be persistent or irreversible.*"[66]

Another 2014 study concluded: "*We suggest that finasteride and dutasteride inhibit 5α-reductase activities and reduce the clearance of glucocorticoids and mineralocorticoids, potentiating insulin resistance, diabetes and vascular disease.*"[67]

Drugs that reduce the levels of DHT are essentially chemically castrating any males who take them. These drugs do not treat the cause of hair loss: they treat one of its symptoms. Do NOT take these drugs for any reason. If you are taking them: stop immediately. Do not underestimate either the unscrupulous greed or influence of multinational corporations. According to a CBS News report in 2011, Merck earns about $400 million a year in revenue from

Propecia. Some people want you to believe that DHT causes hair loss and the only way to stop this is by taking pharmaceuticals.

Closing Thoughts: How to Prevent Your Hair Loss

"As I see it, every day you do one of two things: build health or produce disease in yourself." Adelle Davis

My simple argument is that hair loss signals a chronic issue going on in the body, whether a nutritional, hormonal or toxic imbalance. MPB can be caused by a poor diet, toxin exposure, unhealthy sleep and exercise patterns, elevated stress levels and how we treat our hair. These factors can lead to oxidative stress, inflammation, lipid peroxidation, nutritional deficiencies, hormonal imbalances, metabolic abnormalities, calcification, fibrosis, toxin accumulation and changes in genetic expression, with considerable overlap in these issues. This overall idea is extremely difficult to prove outright. I have presented scientific research backing each argument made but at the end of the day, it is up to you to decide what to believe.

Although the amount of information covered in this book may seem a bit overwhelming, getting started doesn't have to be a complicated process. No transformation can be achieved overnight so take your time with any changes. Hair growth and loss are incredibly complex. I do not have all the answers to your problem. True health is a blend of your own research, listening to intuitions about your body and also the learned advice from your doctor or naturopath. Continue reading and stay well informed. If looking after your health has not been your focus, then you probably need to ask yourself why not. Stop believing that some pill or lotion will solve the problems that your diet and lifestyle have caused.

Eat Real Food

Knowing what you are eating and putting into your body is probably the single most important thing to care about when considering the health of your hair. Eat real food that deeply nourishes the body. Start to cook and prepare your own meals. Try new foods. Your palate changes, so you may like things you didn't enjoy when you were younger. Avoid PUFAs, HFCS, soda, processed foods, fast-food, refined carbohydrates, processed soy, flax, unfiltered tap water, conventionally farmed meat and dairy as well as farmed fish. Eat sea vegetables, fermented foods, soaked nuts and seeds, grass-fed and pastured meat, soaked whole grains, wild fish and lots of fresh fruit and vegetables. Eat more salads. Drink herbal teas, tinctures, full-fat grass-fed raw milk and fresh vegetable juice. Eat organic. Buy food from a local farmer's market or go and pick your own food. Eat food as close to nature as possible and eat what's in season.

Look After Your Hair

Take care of your hair as if it's your most valuable possession. Stop using commercial shampoo and conditioners with toxic chemicals. Stop washing your hair every day. Make your own shampoo and herbal rinses. Massage your scalp every day. Use a wooden comb. Never shower with hot water on your head. Install a water filter. Stop using all other personal-care products with toxic ingredients.

Look After Yourself

Live consciously. Spend more time outside in nature and in the sun. Spend less time in front of a desk, on the phone, looking at a TV or a computer and online. Exercise daily for at least thirty minutes doing something that you enjoy. Make sleep a priority. Simplify your life and reduce your levels of stress. Meditate. Take saunas. Limit your exposure to halogens, synthetic xenoestrogens and heavy metals. Fast for three to ten days, a few times each year. Don't take any pharmaceutical drugs unless absolutely necessary especially antibiotics and antacids. Book an appointment with a naturopathic doctor. Get tested for any nutritional deficiencies or hormonal imbalances you may have. Stop taking any hair loss medication.

Remember: you only get one life. Make the most of it.

Part 7: Appendix
Appendix A: Glossary

5-alpha reductase: The enzyme 5-alpha reductase irreversibly converts testosterone to DHT. You should avoid all 5-alpha reductase inhibitors (finasteride, dutasteride and saw palmetto) as you do not want to inhibit the production of DHT.

ACV: Apple cider vinegar promotes the formation of friendly bacteria in your digestive system. ACV can also be used externally as a conditioner. It has antibacterial and antifungal properties that can heal an itchy, dry scalp.

Adaptogens: Are natural substances that allow the body to adapt to stress. It is believed that adaptogens work by increasing the ability of cells to manufacture and use fuel more efficiently. Some recommended adaptogenic herbs are ashwagandha, He shou wu, mucuna pruriens and holy basil.

Anagen: The growth phase of the hair follicle. This is when the cells in the root of the hair are dividing rapidly and the hair follicle is at its longest, stretching deep into the dermal layer of the skin. Men experiencing hair loss proportionately have less hair in this growth phase. Any factors that increase the anagen phase will result in less hair being lost.

Antioxidants: These protective compounds such as superoxide dismutase, vitamin E, vitamin C and glutathione all inhibit oxidation and reduce free radicals that may lead to cell damage.

Aromatase/Aromatization: This is the process that converts testosterone into oestrogen. This is a natural process and the chief enzyme involved in the conversion is aromatase. As we want to decrease our levels of oestrogen and maintain our levels of testosterone, it is important to prevent aromatization as much as possible.

BPA: Bisphenol-A is often found in various plastics and is a known xenoestrogen. Bisphenol analogs (such as BPS or BPZ) have similar endocrine disruption tendencies.

Calcification: Is the build-up of calcium in body tissue. Calcium is a hardening mineral and so deposits have a negative effect when they accumulate on the scalp and in blood vessels that supply the scalp. This will decrease oxygen and nutrient supply to hair follicles, leading to miniaturization and hair loss.

Catagen: At the end of the growth period of the hair follicle is this short phase. It lasts only a few weeks when growth slows and the hair follicle regresses preparing for a resting phase. The hair growth modulators TGF-beta1 and FGF-5 have been shown to induce this phase.

Dermal Papilla Cells: At the base of the hair follicle is the dermal papilla, containing the blood vessels that deliver nutrients to each follicle. Dermal papilla cells regulate follicle formation and growth.

DHT: Dihydrotestosterone is a male hormone. It is a particularly potent androgen, about five or so times more potent than testosterone.

Endotoxins: Disease-causing bacteria in our gut excrete waste, referred to as endotoxins. These exert a tremendous inflammatory response, increase oestrogen levels, cause the liver to produce more TNF, lower glutathione levels and negatively affect thyroid function.

FGF-5: This is a protein that acts as a signal in initiating the transition of hair follicles from the anagen to the catagen phase. Blocking FGF-5 in the human scalp extends the hair cycle, resulting in a faster growth rate.

Fibrosis: An excess of collagen is called fibrosis and on the scalp may physically impede the growth of hair.

Finasteride: This is an oral, prescription-only medication that lowers DHT levels and can slow the progression of MPB in some men. Marketed as Propecia and Proscar, this drug was originally developed as a treatment for enlarged prostates.

Free testosterone: see Testosterone.

Glutathione: A powerful antioxidant produced in the body or obtained from the diet.

HFCS: High-fructose corn syrup: also known as glucose/fructose. A sweetener made from processing corn.

Insulin Resistance: This is when the cells in the body start resisting or ignoring the signal that insulin is trying to send. Insulin resistance increases the risk of developing type 2 diabetes.

In vitro: In the glass. The term refers to studies that are done with cells or other biological molecules outside their normal biological context.

In vivo: Within the living. The term refers to studies that are done in living organisms.

Lipid Peroxidation: High levels of pro-oxidants lead to lipid peroxidation, a form of oxidative stress that leads to the destruction of unsaturated lipids (fats) in the body.

Lipid Peroxides: One of the chemical products of lipid peroxidation known to cause hair loss.

Microbiome: The flora (bacteria) of the digestive system is collectively known as the microbiome.

Minoxidil: The only MHRA (UK)/FDA (US) approved over-the-counter medication for hair loss. Scientists do not fully understand its efficacy but one working theory is that minoxidil protects the dermal papilla cells from DHT. Another theory is that it widens blood vessels allowing more oxygen, blood and nutrients to the hair follicles. Minoxidil is marketed as Rogaine and Regaine and was originally developed as a treatment for high blood pressure.

MPB: Male Pattern Baldness. It is the most common cause of hair loss in men.

Mycotoxins (mycoestrogens): Mould toxins produced by fungi. There are numerous negative health effects caused by mycotoxins, including elevated oestrogen levels.

Oestrogen (estrogen): Isn't a single hormone but a group of steroid hormones and their bioactive metabolites with oestradiol being the most potent form. In males, oestrogen is synthesized from androgens by the enzyme aromatase.

Oxidative Stress: During times of stress, pro-oxidants (such as ROS, free radicals and peroxides) can increase, resulting in significant damage to cell structures. This is known as oxidative stress. Excessive oxidative stress leads to inflammation.

Phthalates: These known xenoestrogens are used to make plastics soft and flexible. They are also found in personal-care products, laundry detergents and fast food.

Phytic acid: This 'anti-nutrient' is found in many foods including grains, beans, nuts and seeds. Phytic acid interferes with our ability to absorb important nutrients like iron, zinc, calcium and magnesium as well as inhibiting the normal function of digestive enzymes.

Phytoestrogens: These are found in many different plants and potentially can have an oestrogen-like effect on your body. Flax and unfermented soy are the two most potent phytoestrogen-containing foods.

Phytonutrients: Plants contain natural chemical compounds called phytonutrients that are not considered nutrients essential for life. With regard to hair growth, a few may be of particular importance including: quercetin, kaempferol, myricetin, naringenin, apigenin, luteolin, salicin and procyanidins B2 and B3.

Prolactin: Increased levels of this hormone have been shown to promote hair loss and inhibit thyroid function. Prolactin levels are generally elevated in prematurely balding men, and usually caused by stress.

Pro-oxidants: These are compounds that induce oxidation and oxidative stress by generating ROS or by inhibiting antioxidants.

Prostaglandins: These chemicals are part of the body's natural inflammation process and prostaglandin D_2 (PGD_2) has been shown to be increased in the scalps of men with MPB. PGD_2 is known to stimulate calcification and the secretion of prolactin.

PUFAs: Polyunsaturated fatty acids. In excess, PUFAs promote inflammation, reduce testosterone levels, increase aromatase activity and disrupt thyroid function. They also produce lipid peroxides and free radicals that lead to oxidative stress.

ROS: Reactive oxygen species. They are pro-oxidants that induce oxidative damage. Levels of ROS are increased by inflammation and high blood glucose levels and reduced by antioxidants.

Sebum: Sebaceous glands are connected to hair follicles and secrete sebum, an oily substance that lubricates and protects the hair. Excessive sebum production can lead to hair loss.

SHBG: Sex hormone binding globulin. Most testosterone circulating in the blood is bound to SHBG and is essentially 'locked up' and not available for use. The availability of testosterone is therefore influenced by your level of SHBG.

Superoxide dismutase (SOD): This antioxidant enzyme inhibits oxidation and reduces free radicals that may lead to the damage of cells.

Telogen: The final (resting) phase of the hair follicle when growth stops. In a healthy scalp this phase lasts about three to five months and is happening to around 10 percent of hair. Any factors that decrease telogen will result in less hair being lost: and vice versa.

Testosterone: This androgen is mainly produced in the testicles but is also produced in small amounts by the adrenal glands. Most testosterone circulating in your bloodstream is bound to either SHBG or albumin. Only a small fraction of testosterone is unbound to enter a cell and activate its receptor. This is free testosterone. Total testosterone measures all the testosterone that is bound to these two proteins and that which is not.

TGF-beta1: A growth factor important in several biological processes including inflammation and fibrosis. TGF-beta1 levels are related to the progression of MPB and increased levels of prostaglandins.

Total Testosterone: see Testosterone.

VOCs: Volatile organic compounds. Some VOCs such as formaldehyde are dangerous to human health and exposure to them should be avoided.

Xenoestrogens: Foreign oestrogens. They are a sub-category of endocrine disruptors that specifically have oestrogen-like effects. There are three kinds of xenoestrogens: those found in plants (phytoestrogens); those created synthetically in the laboratory (synthetic xenoestrogens); and those found in fungi (mycoestrogens).

ZEA: Zearalenone is the only known mycoestrogen but it is the most common mycotoxin.

Appendix B: Blood Tests

Getting your blood (or urine) tested is very important and will allow you to get a deeper understanding of your state of health, as well as identifying any hormonal or nutritional deficiencies. Not all of these tests are necessary for everybody but each helps to identify possible causes of hair loss. The tests marked with an asterisk (*) are probably a good place to start. Your medical insurance company will not pay for all these tests. Your doctor is also unlikely to order them. You may get some of them as part of a general health check but for many of them you will have to order and pay yourself. Unfortunately reference values for all conventional blood chemistry reports are not standardized or agreed upon as well as the fact that different laboratories use different units (there are plenty of online conversion tables).

Checking that your vitamin and mineral levels are optimum is a sensible precautionary measure. Check your zinc* (preferably toward the high end of the laboratory reference range), copper, iron* (serum ferritin/TIBC), calcium*, and vitamins A, B_6, B_7 (biotin-this test can be expensive), B_9 (folate), B_{12} (if you are deficient, you will probably have elevated homocysteine as a result), C and E.

The ideal range of serum ferritin lies between 40-60 ng/mL. If your ferritin is too high, speak to your doctor about the possibility of donating blood to help reduce your level.

If you are B_{12} deficient then choose a methylcobalamin supplement as this is better absorbed than other types. Preferably use a spray, sublingual or liquid form rather than a tablet.

A blood serum test for magnesium is not accurate so instead order a sublingual epithelial test. Low potassium and calcium are common laboratory signs indicating a magnesium deficiency.

The significance of your hormonal levels is difficult to assess. There are wide normal ranges and it's not easy to predict the accuracy of a single measurement since hormones are affected by daily cycles, seasonal variations and medications. Even so, it is a good idea to check what hormonal issues may be at the root of your problem. Nearly all hormones are measured in relation to testosterone so get tested between 8 to 10 am when your level of testosterone is likely to be highest.

Vitamin D*: Correct blood test for vitamin D status is 25-hydroxycholecaliferol or 25-hydroxyvitamin D (25 OH vitamin D). A level of around 48 ng/mL is preferable. 1,25-dihydroxyvitamin D is NOT the correct test. If you are vitamin D deficient then either spend more time in the sun or take a D3 supplement preferably in liquid form (a daily dose of 2,000 IU).

Total Testosterone*: Range should be between 300-1,080 ng/dL. As base levels vary considerably from man to man it's good to get a reading to have as a reference. Every man is different, so their level of optimal testosterone will be different, too. A target number of 800 ng/dL or higher is what you should ideally be aiming for if you are under 35.

Free Testosterone* (free testosterone index): Optimal range should be 47-244 pg/mL or 9-30 ng/dL. Your percent of free testosterone should be between 1.6-2.9%. A healthy percentage is around 2.5%.

SHBG*: The normal ranges for men are 10-57 nmol/L. Ideally you want to have a reading somewhere around 28-32 nmol/L.

Oestrogen: Oestradiol should be between 22-30 pg/mL. The most accurate test is LC/MS-MS. Elevated levels of oestrogen are typically found in men with increased abdominal obesity. There is no convenient blood test for levels of xenoestrogens. By testing your testosterone, you indirectly measure your levels of oestrogens, so this test is not necessary.

A few tests are required to assess accurately the function of your thyroid gland:
Thyroid-stimulating hormone* (TSH): Optimal range should be between 0.5 to 2.0 mU/L. Many younger men with hair loss have a higher level of TSH suggesting increased cortisol and/or prolactin.
Total T4*; Free T4*; Total T3; Free T3*; Reverse T3(rT3)* and thyroid antibodies*: Readings should be in the middle of your lab's reference range. Elevated reverse T3 usually indicates high levels of stress. Thyroid antibodies should be negative. Free T3 is not part of a regular thyroid panel.

Cortisol/DHEA-S Saliva Test: This measures the levels of the stress hormones DHEA-S and cortisol to help evaluate adrenal function. The preferred method tests four salivary samples and provides an evaluation of how these levels differ throughout the day.

hs-CRP* (not the standard CRP test): Measures C-reactive protein (CRP), a protein that increases in the blood with inflammation. Apart from acute infection/injury, CRP is also an indicator of chronic inflammation. Optimal CRP levels to strive for are under 0.55 mg/L.

Prolactin*: The upper threshold of normal prolactin is about 20 µg/L (425 mIU/L). Ideal levels for men are between 5-10 µg/L. Prolactin strongly indicates oestrogen dominance if it is high. An elevated reading also indicates the thyroid gland is underactive and there are possibly problems with the adrenals.

There is no one test that can directly detect insulin resistance. Laboratory tests most likely to be ordered include:
Fasting plasma glucose (FPG): This test is usually performed while fasting, and determines an impaired response to glucose. A level between 70 and 100 mg/dL is considered normal; above this, your body is showing signs of insulin resistance and diabetes. Ideally, you want to have a reading of less than 85 mg/dL.
Fasting insulin*: You want this reading to be ideally below 5 uIU/mL. A high level of fasting insulin indicates insulin resistance and metabolic syndrome.
Fasting cholesterol* (total triglycerides, HDL and LDL): Total cholesterol should be less than 150 mg/dL. Normal triglyceride levels are less than 150 mg/dL (ideally under 100 mg/dL). An optimal level of HDL cholesterol should be between 55-150 mg/dL. LDL cholesterol should be between 80-120 mg/dL. Insulin resistance and hair loss are both associated with increases in total cholesterol, triglycerides and LDL as well as a decrease in HDL. Elevated cholesterol may indicate a problem with the thyroid.

IGF-1: Is a marker of human growth hormone which is essential to maintaining healthy skin and hair. The test evaluates pituitary function with an optimal range of 200-300 ng/mL. It tends to decrease naturally as we age; however, conditions such as sleep deprivation, diabetes, low thyroid hormone levels, liver disease and insulin resistance can cause levels to decline more rapidly.

Electrolyte Panel: The normal range for CO_2 (bicarbonate) is 22-29 mmol/L (mEq/L) and is used to identify an electrolyte imbalance or acid-base (pH) imbalance. It is typically measured along with sodium, potassium and chloride. These tests can aid in diagnosing adrenal problems.

Lactic acid (lactate): Normal range is 0.5-2.2 mmol/L (4.5-19.8 mg/dL) and is used to test the blood pH for an acid/base imbalance. An elevated level can indicate an infection or disease but can also mean you're not getting enough vitamin B1 (thiamin).

CBC: The complete blood count (full blood count or FBC) is a general blood check for infections in the body that may be leading to complications including hair loss. A low red blood cell count indicates anaemia, often related to low iron, vitamin B_{12} or vitamin B_9 (folate). A low white blood cell count can signal weakened immunity.

Antinuclear Antibodies (ANA): This test is used to determine whether you have an autoimmune disorder such as lupus, a known cause of hair loss.

Luteinizing Hormone (LH) and Follicle Stimulating Hormone (FSH): These two hormones are released from the pituitary gland and stimulate the testes. LH is a hormone associated with testosterone production and an optimal level is between 4-7 mIU/mL. Men with untreated celiac's disease can have moderately high LH levels that usually return to normal upon starting a gluten-free diet. The most common reason for LH deficiency is the use of external androgens such as steroids but an imbalance can be caused by over-exercise, being significantly under or overweight, high stress and using pharmaceutical drugs. The optimal level for FSH is between 2-7 mIU/mL. A high level may mean the testicles are not functioning correctly. Low levels may indicate problems with the pituitary gland.

PTH and calcium: PTH measures the level of parathyroid hormone in the blood. PTH should always be requested with calcium as it is not just the amounts of each that are important. The balance between them is significant and the response of the parathyroid glands to changing concentration of calcium. High blood (serum) calcium concentrations may be due to overproduction of PTH by the parathyroid glands.

Albumin: Hair loss may be caused by lack of protein in the diet. Other situations that may cause a low albumin level include stress, surgery and impaired liver or kidney function. The normal range is 3.5-5.5 g/dL.

If you are having other symptoms such as scalp itching, redness or flaking, you may be suffering from seborrheic dermatitis or another similar condition. You should visit a dermatologist for a scalp examination.

Appendix C: Yoga Poses

Apart from head and shoulder stands, both of which can be quite difficult, there are other simpler yoga poses that increase blood flow to the scalp. These exercises should be done with awareness and synchronized with your breath. Practise every day on an empty stomach for best results.

Shoulder rotation: Sit in a simple cross-legged position with your arms relaxed and hands resting on the knees. Move both shoulders in circles, inhaling as you move them up and back, and exhaling as they move down and forward. Move with slow and relaxed but large circles; ten to twenty rotations backward, then ten to twenty forward. This exercise is a good way to loosen up the shoulder muscles and the upper back. This is a region of tension in men today owing to chronic stress and working at desk jobs.

Neck movement #1: Inhale while looking directly ahead. While exhaling look over your right shoulder as if you are looking behind you. Inhale as you move back to centre and then exhale as you look over your left shoulder. Continue in one fluid motion. 3 to 5 minutes.

Neck movement #2: The chin comes down in the direction of your chest as you exhale. Inhale as you move your head back up to centre and then back so you are looking toward the ceiling. Continue in one fluid motion, moving your head up and down. 3 to 5 minutes.

Neck rotations: Slowly rotate your head in large circles. The right ear moves towards the right shoulder, then allow your head to move forward, chin coming to the chest. Next, the left ear moves towards your left shoulder. Continue each circle in one fluid motion. Inhale when your head is back and exhale as your head is forward. 5 to 10 times clockwise and then anti-clockwise.

Uttanasana (Stand forward bend pose): Stand straight with your feet hip-distance apart. Put your hands on your hips as you inhale deeply and bend forward from the hips. Hang your arms and head freely as you bring your fingertips down to touch the floor. You can bend your knees slightly to avoid any strain in the lower back. Stay in this pose with normal breathing for 3 to 5 minutes. Come out of this pose gently as you inhale deeply and stand back up straight.

Adho Mukha Svanasana (Downward Dog pose): Place your hands and knees on the ground. Inhale as you push your hips up and straighten your legs. Pressing the palms and feet to the ground, straighten your spine. Keep your eyes open with normal breathing for 3 to 5 minutes. To exit, pull down your hips gently and come back to your hands and knees.

Viparita Karani (Legs against the wall pose): Begin by lying on your back with the knees close to your chest. Exhale as you lift your legs up against the wall. The distance from the wall will depend on your height and what feels comfortable. Keep the legs straight and relatively firm as you sink your shoulders and back into the floor. Extend your arms out to the sides, palms facing up. Remain in the pose anywhere from 5 to 10 minutes with relaxed breathing. When coming out of the pose, bend your knees back to the chest, and roll to one side.

Head Hang: Lie flat on your stomach on a bed with your arms flat against your sides. Your head and shoulders are off the edge of the bed. Let your head hang down and completely relax. Hold the posture for 3 to 5 minutes. To return, slowly raise the head and roll to your side.

Appendix D: Websites and References

Here are a few recommended websites that sell organic loose herbs.

In the UK:
Just Ingredients: www.justingredients.co.uk;
Organic Herb Trading Co: www.organicherbtrading.com. Large orders only;
Star Child: www.starchild.co.uk.

In the US:
Banyan Botanicals: www.banyanbotanicals.com;
Mountain Rose Herbs: www.mountainroseherbs.com;
Healing Spirits Herb Farm: www.healingspiritsherbfarm.com;
Pacific Botanicals: www.pacificbotanicals.com. Large orders only.

There were many books and websites that have inspired and helped in the writing of this book. The following list reflects the best of these:

Beauty Detox Solution, The: Kimberly Snyder (Harlequin Books, 2011)
Body Ecology Diet: Recovering Your Health and Rebuilding Your Immunity, The: Donna Gates and Linda Schatz (Body Ecology, 2006)
China Study, The: T. Colin Campbell and Thomas M. Campbell (Benbella Books, 2006)
Colon Health: The Key to a Vibrant Life: Dr Norman Walker (Norwalk Press, 1991)
Complete Book of Chinese Health & Healing: Guarding the Three Treasures, The: Daniel Reid (Shambhala, 2005)
Diet for a New America: John Robbins (HJ Kramer, 1998)
Disease Delusion, The: Dr Jeffrey S. Bland (HarperCollins, 2014)
Estrogeneration: Anthony G. Jay (Pyrimidine Publishing, 2017)
Fresh Vegetable and Fruit Juices: Dr N. W. Walker (Norwalk Press, 1991)
Hair Like a Fox: A Bioenergetic View of Pattern Hair Loss: Danny Roddy (Danny Roddy Weblog LLC, 2013)

Healing with Whole Foods: Oriental Traditions and Modern Nutrition: Paul Pitchford (North Atlantic Books, 1993)

Healthy Gut, Healthy You: The Personalized Plan to Transform Your Health from the Inside Out: Dr Michael Ruscio (The Ruscio Institute, LLC, 2018)

Hormone Diet, The: Natasha Turner (Rodale, 2011)

In Defence of Food: The Myth of Nutrition and the Pleasures of Eating: An Eater's Manifesto: Michael Pollan (Penguin, 2009)

Living Foods for Optimum Health: Brian R.Clement and Theresa Foy Digeronimo (Three Rivers Press, 1998)

Missing Microbes: How the Overuse of Antibiotics is Fueling our Modern Plagues: Martin J. Blaser (Henry Holt and Co, 2014)

Natural Hair Coloring: How to Use Henna and Other Pure Herbal Pigments for Chemical-Free Beauty: Christine Shahin (Storey Publishing, 2016)

Natural Remedies for Low Testosterone: Stephen Harrod Buhner (Healing Arts Press, 2016)

Omnivore's Dilemma, The: The Search for a Perfect Meal in a Fast-Food World: Michael Pollan (Bloomsbury Paperbacks, 2011)

Our Stolen Future: Theo Colborn, Dianne Dumanoski and John Peterson Myers (Plume, 1997)

Primal Body, Primal Mind: Beyond Paleo for Total Health and a Longer Life: Nora Gedgaudas (Healing Arts Press, 2011)

Radical Beauty: How to Transform Yourself from the Inside Out: Deepak Chopra and Kimberley Snyder (Harmony, 2016)

Rosemary Gladstar's Herbal Recipes for Vibrant Health: Rosemary Gladstar (Storey Publishing, 2008)

Sleep Smarter: 21 Essential Strategies to Sleep Your Way to a Better Body, Better Health, and Bigger Success: Shawn Stevenson (Rodale Books, 2016)

Swallow This: Joanna Blythman (Fourth Estate, 2015)

Tao of Detox, The: Daniel Reid (Healing Arts Press, 2006)

Tao of Health, Sex and Longevity, The: Daniel Reid (Prentice Hall, 1989)

Transformational Power of Fasting: Stephen Harrod Buhner (Healing Arts Press, 2012)

Vitamania: How Vitamins Revolutionized the Way We Think About Food: Catherine Price (Penguin Press, 2015)

Whole: Rethinking the Science of Nutrition: T. Colin Campbell and Howard Jacobson (Benbella, 2014)
Wild Fermentation: The Flavor, Nutrition, and Craft of Live-Culture Foods: Sandor Ellix Katz (Chelsea Green Publishing, 2016)

www.anabolicmen.com: information about ways to increase your testosterone levels.
www.dannyroddy.com: extremely informative articles and videos about hair loss.
www.hairbuddha.net: natural ways to help with hair loss.
www.mercola.com: a great natural health website.

References and Notes

Part 1

Amos Barshad, "Is the Age-Old Quest for a Baldness Cure Reaching Its End?" The New Yorker. Published June 7th, 2018.

[2] Koyama T, et al. Eleven pairs of Japanese male twins suggest the role of epigenetic differences in androgenetic alopecia. Eur J Dermatol. 2013;23:113–5.

[3] Gatherwright J, Liu MT, Amirlak B, Gliniak C, Totonchi A, Guyuron B. The contribution of endogenous and exogenous factors to male alopecia: a study of identical twins. Plast Reconstr Surg. 2013;131:794–801.

[4] Known causes of hair loss include excessive sebum, stress, autoimmune disorders, systemic diseases (e.g. psoriasis, thyroid disease, or cancer), dieting and eating disorders, anaemia, heavy metal toxicity, chemotherapy and exposure to radiation, malnourishment, nutritional deficiencies, and severe illness. Many different pharmaceutical prescriptions can also be associated with hair loss including arthritis drugs; blood thinners like heparin and warfarin; epilepsy medication; drugs for ulcers; blood pressure medication (beta-blockers in particular); drugs to lower cholesterol; thyroid medication; anti-inflammatories; drugs that alter the mood, like lithium and Prozac; diet pills with amphetamines; acne medications; antibiotics; anti-fungal medications; tranquilizers; and steroids. A number of infections can contribute to hair loss such as ringworm, folliculitis, piedra, lupus and seborrheic dermatitis. Trauma such as severe burns can also cause permanent hair loss.

[5] 30 Nov 2017: Male-pattern baldness and premature greying are associated with a more than fivefold risk of heart disease before the age of 40 years, according to research presented at the 69th Annual Conference of the Cardiological Society of India.

[6] Ahouansou S, Le Toumelin P, Crickx B, Descamps V. Association of androgenetic alopecia and hypertension. Eur J Dermatol. 2007 May-Jun;17(3):220-2.

[7] Amoretti A, Laydner H, Bergfeld W. Androgenetic alopecia and risk of prostate cancer: a systemic review and meta-analysis. J Am Acad Dermatol. 2013;Jun;68(6):937-43.

[8] Su LH, Chen TH. Association of androgenic alopecia with metabolic syndrome in men: a community-based survey. Br J Dermatol. 2010 Aug;163(2):371-7.

[9] Yang CC, Hsieh FN, Lin LY, Hsu CK, Sheu HM, Chen W. Higher body mass index is associated with greater severity of alopecia in men with male-pattern androgenetic alopecia in Taiwan: A cross-sectional study. J Am Acad Dermatol. 2014;70(2):297-302.

[10] Güngör ES, Güngör S, Zebitay AG. Assessment of semen quality in patients with androgenetic alopecia in an infertility clinic. Dermatologica Sinica. 2016;34(1)10.

[11] Chi W, Wu E, Morgan BA. Dermal papilla cell number specifies hair size, shape and cycling and its reduction causes follicular decline. Development. 2013; Apr;140(8):1676-83.

[12] Lattanand A, Johnson WC. Male Pattern Alopecia A Histopathologic and Histochemical Study. Journal of Cutaneous Pathology Volume 2. Issue 2, August 1975, Pages 58-70.

[13] Williams R, Philpott MP, Kealey T. Metabolism of Freshly Isolated Human Hair Follicles Capable of Hair Elongation: A Glutaminolytic, Aerobic Glycolytic Tissue. Journal of Investigative Dermatology. Volume 100, Issue 6, June 1993, Pages 834-840.

Part 2

Laughlin GA, Barrett-Connor E, Bergstrom J. Low serum testosterone and mortality in older men. J Clin Endocrinol Metab. 2008 Jan;93(1):68-75. Epub 2007 Oct 2.

[2] Urysiak-Czubatka I, Kmieć ML, Broniarczyk-Dyła G. Assessment of the usefulness of dihydrotestosterone in the diagnostics of patients with androgenetic alopecia. Postepy Dermatol Alergol. 2014 Aug; 31(4): 207–215.

[3] Sawaya ME, Price VH. Different levels of 5alpha-reductase type I and II, aromatase, and androgen receptor in hair follicles of women and men with androgenetic alopecia. J Invest Dermatol. 1997;109:296–300.

[4] Vignozzi L, et al. Antiinflammatory effect of androgen receptor activation in human benign prostatic hyperplasia cells. Journal of Endocrinology. 2012; 214(1), 31-43.

[5] Gilliver SC, Ashworth JJ, Mills SJ, Hardman MJ, Ashcroft GS. Androgens modulate the inflammatory response during acute wound healing. Journal of Cell Science. 2006; 119: 722-732.

[6] Norata GD, Tibolla G, Seccomandi PM, Poletti A, Catapano AL. Dihydrotestosterone Decreases Tumor Necrosis Factor-a and Lipopolysaccharide-Induced Inflammatory Response in Human Endothelial Cells. J Clin Endocrinol Metab. 2006 Feb;91(2):546-54.

[7] Gatherwright J, Liu MT, Amirlak B, Gliniak C, Totonchi A, Guyuron B. The contribution of endogenous and exogenous factors to male alopecia: a study of identical twins. Plast Reconstr Surg. 2013;131:794–801.

[8] Stárka L, Cermáková I, Dusková M, Hill M, Dolezal M, Polácek V. Hormonal Profile of Men with Premature Balding. Exp Clin Endocrinol Diabetes. 2004; 112(1): 24-28. "The frequency of subnormal values in SHBG, FSH, testosterone and epitestosterone (but not in free androgen index) was significant in the balding men. A borderline significant trend was recorded with respect to increased levels in 17OH-P and prolactin."

[9] Arias-Santiago S, Gutiérrez-Salmerón MT, Buendía-Eisman A, Girón-Prieto MS, Naranjo-Sintes R. Sex hormone-binding globulin and risk of hyperglycemia in patients with androgenetic alopecia. J Am Acad Dermatol. 2011 Jul;65(1):48-53.

[10] Hawkins VN, et al. Effect of Exercise on Serum Sex Hormones in Men: A 12-Month Randomized Clinical Trial. Med Sci Sports Exerc. 2008 Feb; 40(2): 223–233.

[11] Kelsey TW, Li LQ, Mitchell RT, Whelan A, Anderson RA, Wallace WH. A validated age-related normative model for male total testosterone shows increasing variance but no decline after age 40 years. PLoS One. 2014 Oct 8;9(10).

[12] Perheentupa A, et al. A cohort effect on serum testosterone levels in Finnish men. Eur J Endocrinol. 2013; Jan 17;168(2):227-33.

[13] Ohnemus U, Uenalan M, Inzunza J, Gustafsson JA, Paus R. The hair follicle as an estrogen target and source. Endocr Rev. 2006 Oct;27(6):677-706.

[14] Oh HS, Smart RC. An estrogen receptor pathway regulates the telogen-anagen hair follicle transition and influences epidermal cell proliferation. Proc Natl Acad Sci U S A. 1996 Oct 29; 93(22): 12525–12530.

[15] Schmidt JB, Lindmaier A, Spona J. Hormonal parameters in androgenetic hair loss in the male. Dermatologica. 1991;182(4):214-7.

[16] Rohle D, Wilborn C, Taylor L, Mulligan C, Kreider R, Willoughby D. Effects of eight weeks of an alleged aromatase inhibiting nutritional supplement 6-OXO (androst-4-ene-3,6,17-trione) on serum hormone profiles and clinical safety markers in resistance-trained, eugonadal males. J Int Soc Sports Nutr. 2007; 4: 13.

[17] Nadal A, Alonso-Magdalena P, Soriano S, Quesada I, Ropero AB. The pancreatic beta-cell as a target of estrogens and xenoestrogens: Implications for blood glucose homeostasis and diabetes. Mol Cell Endocrinol. 2009 May 25;304(1-2):63-8.

[18] Thompson LU, Boucher BA, Liu Z, Cotterchio M, Kreiger N. Phytoestrogen content of foods consumed in Canada, including isoflavones, lignans, and coumestan. Nutr Cancer. 2006;54(2):184-201.

[9] Metzler M, Pfeiffer E, Hildebrand AA. Zearalenone and its metabolites as endocrine disrupting chemicals. World mycotoxin journal. 2010 v.3 no.4 pp. 385-401.

[20] Kanora A, Maes D. The role of mycotoxins in pig reproduction : a review. Veterinarni Medicina. 2009; 54(12):565-576.

[21] van Beek N, et al. Thyroid hormones directly alter human hair follicle functions: anagen prolongation and stimulation of both hair matrix keratinocyte proliferation and hair pigmentation. J Clin Endocrinol Metab. 2008 Nov;93(11):4381-8.

[22] Meikle AW. The interrelationships between thyroid dysfunction and hypogonadism in men and boys. Thyroid. 2004;14 Suppl 1:S17-25.

[23] Mancini A, et al. Thyroid Hormones, Oxidative Stress, and Inflammation. Mediators of Inflammation. Volume 2016, Article ID 6757154, 12 pages.

[24] Sanke S, Chander R, Jain A, Garg T, Yadav P. A Comparison of the Hormonal Profile of Early Androgenetic Alopecia in Men With the Phenotypic Equivalent of Polycystic Ovarian Syndrome in Women. JAMA Dermatol. 2016 Sep 1;152(9):986-91.

[25] Foitzik K, Langan EA, Paus R. Prolactin and the Skin: A Dermatological Perspective on an Ancient Pleiotropic Peptide Hormone. Journal of Investigative Dermatology. Volume 129, Issue 5, May 2009, Pages 1071-1087.

[26] Daimon, M, et al. Association between serum prolactin levels and insulin resistance in non-diabetic men. PLoS One. 2017; 12(4): e0175204.

[27] Zhang, H et al. Effects of pterostilbene on treating hyperprolactinemia and related mechanisms. American journal of translational research. vol. 8,7 3049-55. 15 Jul. 2016.

[28] Thom E. Stress and the Hair Growth Cycle: Cortisol-Induced Hair Growth Disruption. J Drugs Dermatol. 2016 Aug 1;15(8):1001-4.

[29] Svenstrup, B., et al. Comparison of the effect of cortisol on aromatase activity and androgen metabolism in two human fibroblast cell lines derived from the same individual. J Steroid Biochem. 1990 May;35(6):679-87.

[30] Starka L, Duskova M, Cermakova I, Vrbiková J, Hill M. Premature androgenic alopecia and insulin resistance. Male equivalent of polycystic ovary syndrome? Endocr Regul. 2005 Dec;39(4):127-31.

[31] Patterson E, Wall R, Fitzgerald GF, Ross RP, Stanton C. Health implications of high dietary omega-6 polyunsaturated Fatty acids. J Nutr Metab. 2012;2012:539426.

[32] Pengsalae N, Tanglertsampan C, Phichawong T, Lee S. Association of early-onset androgenetic alopecia and metabolic syndrome in Thai men: a case-control study. J. Med. Assoc. Thai. 96(8), 947–951 (2013).

[33] Behrangi E, et al. Association of Androgenic Alopecia with Metabolic Syndrome. Ann Med Health Sci Res. 2018;8:91-93.

[34] Cannarella R, et al. Glycolipid and Hormonal Profiles in Young Men with Early-Onset Androgenic Alopecia: A meta-analysis. Scientific Reports 7. 2017; 7801.

[35] Trieu N, Eslick GD. Alopecia and its association with coronary heart disease and cardiovascular risk factors: a meta-analysis. Int J Cardiol. 2014 Oct 20;176(3):687-95.

[36] Keane KN, Cruzat VF, Carlessi R, Homem de Bittencourt, Jr. PI, Newsholme P. Molecular Events Linking Oxidative Stress and Inflammation to Insulin Resistance and β-Cell Dysfunction. Oxid Med Cell Longev. 2015: 181643.

[37] Hurrle S, Hsu WH. The etiology of oxidative stress in insulin resistance. Biomed J. 2017 Oct; 40(5): 257–262.

[38] Mishra S, Mishra BB. Study of Lipid Peroxidation, Nitric Oxide End Product, and Trace Element Status in Type 2 Diabetes Mellitus with and without Complications. Int J Appl Basic Med Res. 2017 Apr-Jun; 7(2): 88–93.

[39] Caricilli AM, Saad MJA. Nutrients. The Role of Gut Microbiota on Insulin Resistance. 2013 Mar; 5(3): 829–851.

[40] Upton JH, et al. Oxidative stress-associated senescence in dermal papilla cells of men with androgenetic alopecia. J Invest Dermatol. 2015 May;135(5):1244-1252.

[41] Wang L, et al. Oxidative stress and substance P mediate psychological stress-induced autophagy and delay of hair growth in mice. Arch Dermatol Res. 2015 Mar;307(2):171-81.

[42] Shin H, et al. Induction of transforming growth factor-beta 1 by androgen is mediated by reactive oxygen species in hair follicle dermal papilla cells. BMB Rep. 2013 Sep;46(9):460-4.

[43] Gatherwright J, et al. The contribution of endogenous and exogenous factors to male alopecia: a study of identical twins. Plast Reconstr Surg. 2013;131:794–801.

[44] Naito A, Midorikawa T, Yoshino T, Ohdera M. Lipid peroxides induce early onset of catagen phase in murine hair cycles. Int J Mol Med. 2008 Dec;22(6):725-9.

[45] Mylonas C, Kouretas D. Lipid peroxidation and tissue damage. In Vivo. 1999 May-Jun;13(3):295-309.

[46] Haggag Mel-S, Elsanhoty RM, Ramadan MF. Impact of dietary oils and fats on lipid peroxidation in liver and blood of albino rats. Asian Pac J Trop Biomed. 2014 Jan; 4(1): 52–58.

[47] El-Domyati M, Attia S, Saleh F, Abdel-Wahab H. Androgenetic alopecia in males: a histopathological and ultrastructural study. J Cosmet Dermatol. 2009 Jun;8(2):83-91.

[48] Sakr FM, Gado AM, Mohammed HR, Adam AN. Preparation and evaluation of a multimodal minoxidil microemulsion versus minoxidil alone in the treatment of androgenic alopecia of mixed etiology: a pilot study. Drug Des Devel Ther. 2013; 7: 413–423.

[49] Sueki H, Stoudemayer T, Kligman AM, Murphy GF. Quantitative and ultrastructural analysis of inflammatory infiltrates in male pattern alopecia. Acta Derm Venereol. 1999 Sep;79(5):347-50.

[50] Young JW, Conte ET, Leavitt ML, Nafz MA, Schroeter AL. Cutaneous immunopathology of androgenetic alopecia. J Am Osteopath Assoc. 1991 Aug;91(8):765-71.

[51] Lattanand A, Johnson WC. Male Pattern Alopecia A Histopathologic and Histochemical Study. Journal of Cutaneous Pathology Volume 2. Issue 2, August 1975, Pages 58-70.

[52] Zouboulis CC. Acne and sebaceous gland function. Clin Dermatol. 2004 Sep-Oct;22(5):360-6.

[53] Jayaraman A, Lent-Schochet D, Pike CJ. Diet-induced obesity and low testosterone increase neuroinflammation and impair neural function. J Neuroinflammation. 2014 Sep 16;11:162.

[54] Tsilidis KK, et al. Association between endogenous sex steroid hormones and inflammatory biomarkers in US men. Andrology. 2013 Nov;1(6):919-28.

[55] Gaschler MM, Stockwell BR. Lipid peroxidation in cell death. Biochem Biophys Res Commun. 2017 Jan 15;482(3):419-425.

[56] Haribabu A, et al. Evaluation of protein oxidation and its association with lipid peroxidation and thyrotropin levels in overt and subclinical hypothyroidism. Endocrine. 2013;44(1):152–157.

[57] L. Montenegro et al., "Nonsteroidal Anti-Inflammatory Drug Induced Damage on Lower Gastro-Intestinal Tract: Is There an Involvement of Microbiota?" Curr Drug Saf. 2014;9(3):196-204.

[58] Koshihara Y, Kawamura M. Prostaglandin D2 stimulates calcification of human osteoblastic cells. Biochem Biophys Res Commun. 1989 Mar 31;159(3):1206-12.

[59] Garza LA, et al. Prostaglandin D2 inhibits hair growth and is elevated in bald scalp of men with androgenetic alopecia. Sci Transl Med. 2012 Mar 21;4(126):126ra34.

[60] Jeong KH, Jung JH, Kim JE, Kang H. Prostaglandin D2-Mediated DP2 and AKT Signal Regulate the Activation of Androgen Receptors in Human Dermal Papilla Cells. Int J Mol Sci. 2018 Feb; 19(2): 556.

[61] Toma I, McCaffrey TA. Transforming growth factor-β and atherosclerosis: interwoven atherogenic and atheroprotective aspects. Cell Tissue Res. 2012 Jan; 347(1): 155–175.

[62] Foitzik K, et al. Control of murine hair follicle regression (catagen) by TGF-beta1 in vivo. FASEB J. 2000 Apr;14(5):752-60.

[63] Liu RM, Desai LP. Reciprocal regulation of TGF-β and reactive oxygen species: A perverse cycle for fibrosis. Redox Biol. 2015 Dec; 6: 565–577.

[64] Lucia MS, Sporn MB, Roberts AB, Stewart LV, Danielpour D. The role of transforming growth factor-beta1, -beta2, and -beta3 in androgen-responsive growth of NRP-152 rat prostatic epithelial cells. J Cell Physiol. 1998 May;175(2):184-92.

[65] Philpott MP, Sanders DA, Bowen J, Kealey T. Effects of interleukins, colony-stimulating factor and tumour necrosis factor on human hair follicle growth in vitro: a possible role for interleukin-1 and tumour necrosis factor-alpha in alopecia areata. Br J Dermatol. 1996 Dec;135(6):942-8.

[66] Bianchi, VE. The Anti-Inflammatory Effects of Testosterone. J Endocr Soc. 2019 Jan 1; 3(1): 91–107.

[67] Poth M, Tseng YC, Wartofsky L. Inhibition of TSH activation of human cultured thyroid cells by tumor necrosis factor: an explanation for decreased thyroid function in systemic illness? Thyroid. 1991 Summer;1(3):235-40.

[68] Gonzalez Y, et al. High glucose concentrations induce TNF-α production through the down-regulation of CD33 in primary human monocytes. BMC Immunol. 2012 Apr 14;13:19.

[69] Traish A, Bolanos J, Nair S, Saad F, Morgentaler A. Do Androgens Modulate the Pathophysiological Pathways of Inflammation? Appraising the Contemporary Evidence. J Clin Med. 2018 Dec 14;7(12).

[70] Itoh Y, et al. Dihydrotestosterone inhibits tumor necrosis factor alpha induced interleukin-1alpha mRNA expression in rheumatoid fibroblast-like synovial cells. Biol Pharm Bull. 2007 Jun;30(6):1140-3.

[71] Ota Y, Saitoh Y, Suzuki S, Ozawa K, Kawano M, Imamura T. Fibroblast growth factor 5 inhibits hair growth by blocking dermal papilla cell activation. Biochem Biophys Res Commun. 2002 Jan 11;290(1):169-76.

[72] Wester RC, Maibach HI, Guy RH, Novak E. Minoxidil stimulates cutaneous blood flow in human balding scalps: pharmacodynamics measured by laser Doppler velocimetry and photopulse plethysmography. J, Invest Dermatol 1984;82:515-7.

[73] Goldman BE, Fisher DM, Ringler SL. Transcutaneous PO2 of the scalp in male pattern baldness: a new piece to the puzzle. Plast Reconstr Surg. 1996 May;97(6):1109-16; discussion 1117.

[74] Klemp P, Peters K, Hansted B. Subcutaneous blood flow in early male pattern baldness. J Invest Dermatol. 1989 May;92(5):725-6.

[75] Freund BJ, Schwartz M. Treatment of male pattern baldness with botulinum toxin: a pilot study. Plast Reconstr Surg. 2010 Nov;126(5):246e-248e.

[76] Singh S, Neema S, Vasudevan B. A Pilot Study to Evaluate Effectiveness of Botulinum Toxin in Treatment of Androgenetic Alopecia in Males. J Cutan Aesthet Surg. 2017 Jul-Sep; 10(3): 163–167.

[77] Yoo HG, et al. Perifollicular fibrosis: pathogenetic role in androgenetic alopecia. Biol Pharm Bull. 2006 Jun;29(6):1246-50.

[78] Won CH, et al. Dermal fibrosis in male pattern hair loss: a suggestive implication of mast cells. Arch Dermatol Res. 2008 Mar;300(3):147-52.

[79] Jaworsky C, Kligman AM, Murphy GF. Characterization of inflammatory infiltrates in male pattern alopecia: implications for pathogenesis. Br J Dermatol. 1992 Sep;127(3):239-46.

[80] Hoelzel, F. Baldness and Calcification of the "Ivory Dome." JAMA. 1942;119(12):968. doi:10.1001/jama.1942.

[81] Pechlivanis S, et al. Male-pattern baldness and incident coronary heart disease and risk factors in the Heinz Nixdorf Recall Study. PLoS ONE. 2019;14(11): e0225521.

[82] Ahouansou S, Le Toumelin P, Crickx B, Descamps V. Association of androgenetic alopecia and hypertension. Eur J Dermatol. 2007 May-Jun;17(3):220-2.

[83] Li Y, Berenji GR, Shaba WF, Tafti B, Yevdayev E, Dadparvar S. Association of vascular fluoride uptake with vascular calcification and coronary artery disease. Nucl Med Commun. 2012 Jan;33(1):14-20.

[84] Zhang Y, et al. Thyroid hormones and coronary artery calcification in euthyroid men and women. Arterioscler Thromb Vasc Biol. 2014 Sep;34(9):2128-34.

[85] Park B, Kim MH, Cha CK, Lee YJ, Kim KC. High Calcium-Magnesium Ratio in Hair Is Associated with Coronary Artery Calcification in Middle-Aged and Elderly Individuals. Biol Trace Elem Res. 2017 Sep;179(1):52-58.

Part 3

Kimmons J, Gillespie C, Seymour J, Serdula M, Blanck HM. Fruit and vegetable intake among adolescents and adults in the United States: percentage meeting individualized recommendations. Medscape J Med. 2009;11(1):26.

[2] Misner, B. Food Alone May Not Provide Sufficient Micronutrients for Preventing Deficiency. J Int Soc Sports Nutr. 2006; 3(1): 51–55.

[3] The National Health and Nutrition Examination Survey, 2011.

[4] Gowda D, Premalatha V, Imtiyaz DB. Prevalence of Nutritional Deficiencies in Hair Loss among Indian Participants: Results of a Cross-sectional Study. Int J Trichology. 2017 Jul-Sep; 9(3): 101–104.

[5] Kil MS, Kim CW, Kim SS. Analysis of Serum Zinc and Copper Concentrations in Hair Loss. Ann Dermatol. 2013 Nov; 25(4): 405–409.

[6] Jin W, Zhu Z, Wu S, Zhang X, Zhou X. Determination of zinc, copper, iron and manganese contents in hair for MPA patients and healthy men. Guang Pu Xue Yu Guang Pu Fen Xi. 1998 Feb;18(1):91-3.

[7] Rajput R. The Concept of Cyclical Nutritional Therapy for Hair Growth which can be Applied for Wellness. J Nutr Food Sci 2017, 7:4

[8] Rutkowski M, Grzegorczyk K. Adverse effects of antioxidative vitamins. Int J Occup Med Environ Health. 2012 Jun;25(2):105-21.

[9] Guo EL, Katta R. Diet and hair loss: effects of nutrient deficiency and supplement use. Dermatol Pract Concept. 2017 Jan; 7(1): 1–10.

[10] Anderson JJ, et al. Calcium Intake From Diet and Supplements and the Risk of Coronary Artery Calcification and its Progression Among Older Adults: 10-Year Follow-up of the Multi-Ethnic Study of Atherosclerosis (MESA). J Am Heart Assoc. 2016 Oct 11;5(10).

[11] Davis DR, Epp MD, Riordan HD. Changes in USDA food composition data for 43 garden crops, 1950 to 1999. J Am Coll Nutr. 2004 Dec;23(6):669-82.

[12] Mayer, A-M. Historical changes in the mineral content of fruits and vegetables. British Food Journal. 1997;99/6:207–211.

[13] Worthington V. Nutritional quality of organic versus conventional fruits, vegetables, and grains. J Altern Complement Med. 2001 Apr;7(2):161-73.

[14] Barański M, et al. Higher antioxidant and lower cadmium concentrations and lower incidence of pesticide residues in organically grown crops: a systematic literature review and meta-analyses. Br J Nutr. 2014 Sep 14;112(5):794-811.

[15] Fan W, et al. Herbicide atrazine activates SF-1 by direct affinity and concomitant co-activators recruitments to induce aromatase expression via promoter II. Biochem Biophys Res Commun. 2007 Apr 20;355(4):1012-8.

[16] Brandão Néto J, et al. Zinc: an inhibitor of prolactin (PRL) secretion in humans. Horm Metab Res. 1989 Apr;21(4):203-6.

[17] Betsy A, Binitha M, Sarita S. Zinc Deficiency Associated with Hypothyroidism: An Overlooked Cause of Severe Alopecia. Int J Trichology. 2013 Jan-Mar; 5(1): 40–42.

[18] Prasad AS, Mantzoros CS, Beck FW, Hess JW, Brewer GJ. Zinc status and serum testosterone levels of healthy adults. Nutrition. 1996 May;12(5):344-8.

[19] Om AS, Chung KW. Dietary zinc deficiency alters 5 alpha-reduction and aromatization of testosterone and androgen and estrogen receptors in rat liver. J Nutr. 1996 Apr;126(4):842-8.

[20] Ruz M, et al. Single and multiple selenium-zinc-iodine deficiencies affect rat thyroid metabolism and ultrastructure. J Nutr. 1999 Jan;129(1):174-80.

[21] King DE, Mainous AG 3rd, Geesey ME, Woolson RF. Dietary magnesium and C-reactive protein levels. J Am Coll Nutr. 2005 Jun;24(3):166-71.

[22] ter Braake AD, Tinnemans PT, Shanahan CM, Hoenderop JGJ, de Baaij JHF. Magnesium prevents vascular calcification in vitro by inhibition of hydroxyapatite crystal formation. Sci Rep. 2018; 8: 2069.

[23] Park B, Kim MH, Cha CK, Lee YJ, Kim KC. High Calcium-Magnesium Ratio in Hair Is Associated with Coronary Artery Calcification in Middle-Aged and Elderly Individuals. Biol Trace Elem Res. 2017 Sep;179(1):52-58.

[24] van den Broek FA, Beynen AC. The influence of dietary phosphorus and magnesium concentrations on the calcium content of heart and kidneys of DBA/2 and NMRI mice. Lab Anim. 1998 Oct;32(4):483-91.

[25] Cinar V, Polat Y, Baltaci AK, Mogulkoc R. Effects of magnesium supplementation on testosterone levels of athletes and sedentary subjects at rest and after exhaustion. Biol Trace Elem Res. 2011 Apr;140(1):18-23.

[26] Dibaba DT, Xun P, He K. Dietary Magnesium Intake is Inversely Associated with Serum C-reactive Protein Levels: Meta-analysis and Systematic Review. Eur J Clin Nutr. 2014 Apr; 68(4): 510–516.

[27] Calvo MS, Moshfegh AJ, Tucker KL. Assessing the Health Impact of Phosphorus in the Food Supply: Issues and Considerations. Adv Nutr. 2014 Jan; 5(1): 104–113.

[28] Adeney KL, et al. Association of serum phosphate with vascular and valvular calcification in moderate CKD. J Am Soc Nephrol. 2009 Feb;20(2):381-7.

[29] Park SY, Na SY, Kim JH, Cho S, Lee JH. Iron Plays a Certain Role in Patterned Hair Loss. J Korean Med Sci. 2013 Jun; 28(6): 934–938.

[30] Britton RS, Bacon BR, Recknagel RO. Lipid peroxidation and associated hepatic organelle dysfunction in iron overload. Chem Phys Lipids. 1987 Nov-Dec;45(2-4):207-39.

[31] Omara FO, Blakley BR. Vitamin E is protective against iron toxicity and iron-induced hepatic vitamin E depletion in mice. J Nutr. 1993 Oct;123(10):1649-55.

[32] Safarinejad MR, Safarinejad S. Efficacy of selenium and/or N-acetyl-cysteine for improving semen parameters in infertile men: a double-blind, placebo controlled, randomized study. J Urol. 2009 Feb;181(2):741-51.

[33] Ralston NV, Raymond LJ. Dietary selenium's protective effects against methylmercury toxicity. Toxicology. 2010 Nov 28;278(1):112-23.

[34] Mutter J. Is dental amalgam safe for humans? The opinion of the scientific committee of the European Commission. J Occup Med Toxicol. 2011 Jan 13;6(1):2.

[35] Wehr E, Pilz S, Boehm BO, März W, Obermayer-Pietsch B. Association of vitamin D status with serum androgen levels in men. Clin Endocrinol (Oxf). 2010 Aug;73(2):243-8.

[36] Halicka HD, et al. Attenuation of constitutive DNA damage signaling by 1,25-dihydroxyvitamin D3. Aging (Albany NY). 2012 Apr;4(4):270-8.

[37] Gominak SC. Vitamin D deficiency changes the intestinal microbiome reducing B vitamin production in the gut. The resulting lack of pantothenic acid adversely affects the immune system, producing a "pro-inflammatory" state associated with atherosclerosis and autoimmunity. Med Hypotheses. 2016 Sep;94:103-7.

[38] Aoi N, et al. 1α,25-dihydroxyvitamin D3 modulates the hair-inductive capacity of dermal papilla cells: therapeutic potential for hair regeneration. Stem Cells Transl Med. 2012 Aug;1(8):615-26.

[39] Gade VKV, Mony A, Munisamy M, Chandrashekar L, Rajappa M. An investigation of vitamin D status in alopecia areata. Clin Exp Med. 2018 Nov;18(4):577-584. "Our results suggest significant systemic inflammation and vitamin D deficiency in alopecia areata, more so with increasing disease severity."

[40] Rasheed H, et al. Serum ferritin and vitamin D in female hair loss: do they play a role? Skin Pharmacol Physiol. 2013;26(2):101-7.

[41] Nayak K, Garg A, Mithra P, Manjrekar P. Serum Vitamin D3 Levels and Diffuse Hair Fall among the Student Population in South India: A Case–Control Study. Int J Trichology. 2016 Oct-Dec; 8(4): 160–164.

[42] Ginde AA, Liu MC, Camargo CA Jr. Demographic differences and trends of vitamin D insufficiency in the US population, 1988-2004. Arch Intern Med. 2009 Mar 23;169(6):626-32.

[43] Umeda F, Kato K, Muta K, Ibayashi H. Effect of vitamin E on function of pituitary-gonadal axis in male rats and human subjects. Endocrinol Jpn. 1982 Jun;29(3):287-92.

[44] Yeksan M, et al. Effect of vitamin E therapy on sexual functions of uremic patients in hemodialysis. Int J Artif Organs. 1992 Nov;15(11):648-52.

[45] Beoy LA, Woei WJ, Hay YK. Effects of Tocotrienol Supplementation on Hair Growth in Human Volunteers. Trop Life Sci Res. 2010 Dec; 21(2): 91–99.

[46] Naziroglu M, Kokcam I. Antioxidants and lipid peroxidation status in the blood of patients with alopecia. Cell Biochem Funct. 2000 Sep;18(3):169-73.

[47] Maggio M, et al. Relationship between Carotenoids, Retinol, and Oestradiol Levels in Older Women. Nutrients. 2015 Aug; 7(8): 6506–6519.

[48] Krajcovicová-Kudláčková M, Pauková V, Baceková M, Dusinská M. Lipid peroxidation in relation to vitamin C and vitamin E levels. Cent Eur J Public Health. 2004 Mar;12(1):46-8.

[49] Kwack MH, et al. l-Ascorbic acid 2-phosphate promotes elongation of hair shafts via the secretion of insulin-like growth factor-1 from dermal papilla cells through phosphatidylinositol 3-kinase. Br J Dermatol. 2009 Jun;160(6):1157-62.

[50] Flore R, et al. Something more to say about calcium homeostasis: the role of vitamin K2 in vascular calcification and osteoporosis. Eur Rev Med Pharmacol Sci. 2013 Sep;17(18):2433-40.

[51] Otsuka M, et al. Vitamin K2 binds 17beta-hydroxysteroid dehydrogenase 4 and modulates estrogen metabolism. Life Sci. 2005 Apr 8;76(21):2473-82.

[52] Hou YJ, et al. Mycotoxin-containing diet causes oxidative stress in the mouse. PLoS One. 2013;8(3):e60374.

[53] Yamaguti PM, et al. Effects of Single Exposure of Sodium Fluoride on Lipid Peroxidation and Antioxidant Enzymes in Salivary Glands of Rats. Oxid Med Cell Longev. 2013; 2013: 674593.

[54] Prie BE, Iosif L, Tivig I, Stoian I, Giurcaneanu C. Oxidative stress in androgenetic alopecia. J Med Life. 2016 Jan-Mar; 9(1): 79–83.

[55] Krishnamurthy P, Wadhwani A . Antioxidant enzymes and human health. Antioxidant enzyme, Rijeka, Croatia: InTech; 2012: Pp. 3-18.

[56] Wikramanayake TC, et al. Prevention and treatment of alopecia areata with quercetin in the C3H/HeJ mouse model. Cell Stress Chaperones. 2012 Mar;17(2):267-74.

[57] Yao L, et al. Quercetin, Inflammation and Immunity. Nutrients. 2016 Mar; 8(3): 167.

[58] Sanderson JT, et al. Induction and inhibition of aromatase (CYP19) activity by natural and synthetic flavonoid compounds in H295R human adrenocortical carcinoma cells. Toxicol Sci. 2004 Nov;82(1):70-9.

[59] Taira N, Nguyen BC, Tawata S. Hair Growth Promoting and Anticancer Effects of p21-activated kinase 1 (PAK1) Inhibitors Isolated from Different Parts of *Alpinia zerumbet*. Molecules. 2017 Jan; 22(1): 132.

[60] Zhuang Z, Ye G, Huang B. Kaempferol Alleviates the Interleukin-1β-Induced Inflammation in Rat Osteoarthritis Chondrocytes via Suppression of NF-κB. Med Sci Monit. 2017 Aug 14;23:3925-3931.

[61] Zhang MJ, et al. Chemopreventive effect of Myricetin, a natural occurring compound, on colonic chronic inflammation and inflammation-driven tumorigenesis in mice. Biomed Pharmacother. 2018 Jan;97:1131-1137.

[62] Bennett CJ, et al. Potential therapeutic antioxidants that combine the radical scavenging ability of myricetin and the lipophilic chain of vitamin E to effectively inhibit microsomal lipid peroxidation. Bioorg Med Chem. 2004 May 1;12(9):2079-98.

[63] Ong KC, Khoo HE. Effects of myricetin on glycemia and glycogen metabolism in diabetic rats. Life Sci. 2000 Aug 25;67(14):1695-705.

[64] Alka Madaan, et al. *In vitro* Hair Growth Promoting Effects of Naringenin and Hesperetin on Human Dermal Papilla Cells and Keratinocytes. American Journal of Dermatology and Venereology. 2017, 6(3): 51-57.

[65] Hernández-Aquino E, Muriel P. Beneficial effects of naringenin in liver diseases: Molecular mechanisms. World J Gastroenterol. 2018 Apr 28; 24(16): 1679–1707.

[66] Huh S, et al. A cell-based system for screening hair growth-promoting agents. Arch Dermatol Res. 2009 Jun;301(5):381-5.

[67] Jeong HJ, Shin YG, Kim IH, Pezzuto JM. Inhibition of aromatase activity by flavonoids. Arch Pharm Res. 1999 Jun;22(3):309-12.

[68] Aziz N, Kim MY, Cho JY. Anti-inflammatory effects of luteolin: A review of in vitro, in vivo, and in silico studies. J Ethnopharmacol. 2018 Oct 28;225:342-358.

[69] Li F, et al. Coadministrating luteolin minimizes the side effects of the aromatase inhibitor letrozole. J Pharmacol Exp Ther. 2014 Nov;351(2):270-7.

[70] Shirley D, McHale C, Gomez G. Resveratrol preferentially inhibits IgE-dependent PGD2 biosynthesis but enhances TNF production from human skin mast cells. Biochim Biophys Acta. 2016 Apr;1860(4):678-85

[71] Salehi B, et al. Resveratrol: A Double-Edged Sword in Health Benefits. Biomedicines. 2018 Sep; 6(3):91.

[72] Wang Y, Lee KW, Chan FL, Chen S, Leung LK. The red wine polyphenol resveratrol displays bilevel inhibition on aromatase in breast cancer cells. Toxicol Sci. 2006 Jul;92(1):71-7.

[73] Dündar Y, et al. Synthesis and biological evaluation of the salicylamide and salicylic acid derivatives as anti-estrogen agents. Med Chem. 2012 May;8(3):481-90.

[74] Randjelovic P, et al. The Beneficial Biological Properties of Salicylic Acid. Acta Facultatis Medicae Naissensis. 2015 Dec;32(4):259-265.

[75] Kamimura A, Takahashi T. Procyanidin B-2, extracted from apples, promotes hair growth: a laboratory study. Br J Dermatol. 2002 Jan;146(1):41-51.

[76] Eng ET, et al. Suppression of estrogen biosynthesis by procyanidin dimers in red wine and grape seeds. Cancer Res. 2003 Dec 1;63(23):8516-22.

[77] Kamimura A, Takahashi T. Procyanidin B-3, isolated from barley and identified as a hair-growth stimulant, has the potential to counteract inhibitory regulation by TGF-beta1. Exp Dermatol. 2002 Dec;11(6):532-41.

[78] Oizumi Y, Mohri Y, Hirota M, Makabe H. Synthesis of procyanidin B3 and its anti-inflammatory activity. the effect of 4-alkoxy group of catechin electrophile in the Yb(OTf)(3)-catalyzed condensation with catechin nucleophile. J Org Chem. 2010 Jul 16;75(14):4884-6.

[79] Barański M, et al. Higher antioxidant and lower cadmium concentrations and lower incidence of pesticide residues in organically grown crops: a systematic literature review and meta-analyses. Br J Nutr. 2014 Sep 14;112(5):794-811.

[80] Rossella Cannarella, et al. Increased DHEAS and Decreased Total Testosterone Serum Levels in a Subset of Men with Early-Onset Androgenetic Alopecia: Does a Male PCOS-Equivalent Exist? Int J Endocrinol. 2020; 2020: 1942126.

[81] Pitts RL. Serum elevation of dehydroepiandrosterone sulfate associated with male pattern baldness in young men. J Am Acad Dermatol. 1987 Mar;16(3 Pt 1):571-3.

[82] Schmidt JB, Lindmaier A, Spona J. Hormonal parameters in androgenetic hair loss in the male. Dermatologica. 1991;182(4):214-7.

[83] El-Esawy FM, El-Rahman SH. Androgenetic alopecia as an early marker for hypertension. Egypt J Dermatol Venerol. 2013;33:63-6.

[84] Suez J, Korem T, Zilberman-Schapira G, Segal E, Elinavra E. Non-caloric artificial sweeteners and the microbiome: findings and challenges. Gut Microbes. 2015; 6(2): 149–155.

[85] Fernández MF, et al. Breast Cancer and Its Relationship with the Microbiota. Int J Environ Res Public Health. 2018 Aug 14;15(8). pii: E1747

[86] Ding S, Lund PK. Role of intestinal inflammation as an early event in obesity and insulin resistance. Curr Opin Clin Nutr Metab Care. 2011 Jul; 14(4): 328–333.

[87] Le Chatelier E, et al. Richness of human gut microbiome correlates with metabolic markers. Nature. 2013 Aug 29;500(7464):541-6.

[88] Bailey MT, et al. Exposure to a social stressor alters the structure of the intestinal microbiota: implications for stressor-induced immunomodulation. Brain Behav Immun. 2011 Mar;25(3):397-407.

[89] Vakharia K, Hinson JP. Lipopolysaccharide directly stimulates cortisol secretion by human adrenal cells by a cyclooxygenase-dependent mechanism. Endocrinology. 2005 Mar;146(3):1398-402.

[90] Christeff N, et al. Effect of the aromatase inhibitor, 4 hydroxyandrostenedione, on the endotoxin-induced changes in steroid hormones in male rats. Life Sci. 1992;50(19):1459-68.

[91] Zhu Y, Carvey PM, Ling Z. Altered glutathione homeostasis in animals prenatally exposed to lipopolysaccharide. Neurochem Int. 2007 Mar; 50(4): 671–680.

[92] Boelen A, et al. Interleukin-18, a proinflammatory cytokine, contributes to the pathogenesis of non-thyroidal illness mainly via the central part of the hypothalamus-pituitary-thyroid axis. Eur J Endocrinol. 2004 Oct;151(4):497-502.

[93] Tremellen K, et al. Endotoxin-initiated inflammation reduces testosterone production in men of reproductive age. Am J Physiol Endocrinol Metab. 2018 Mar 1;314(3):E206-E213.

[94] Ferrocino I, et al. Fecal Microbiota in Healthy Subjects Following Omnivore, Vegetarian and Vegan Diets: Culturable Populations and rRNA DGGE Profiling. PLoS One. 2015 Jun 2;10(6):e0128669.

Part 4

Di Noia J. Defining Powerhouse Fruits and Vegetables: A Nutrient Density Approach. Prev Chronic Dis 2014;11:130390.

[2] Gülçin I, Küfrevioglu OI, Oktay M, Büyükokuroglu ME. Antioxidant, antimicrobial, antiulcer and analgesic activities of nettle (Urtica dioica L.). J Ethnopharmacol. 2004 Feb;90(2-3):205-15.

[3] Jo Robinson, "Breeding the Nutrition Out of Our Food" New York Times. Published May 25th, 2013.

[4] De Santi M, et al. Inhibition of Testosterone Aromatization by the Indole-3-carbinol Derivative CTet in CYP19A1-overexpressing MCF-7 Breast Cancer Cells. Anticancer Agents Med Chem. 2015;15(7):896-904.

[5] Chen XL, Dodd G, Kunsch C. Sulforaphane inhibits TNF-alpha-induced activation of p38 MAP kinase and VCAM-1 and MCP-1 expression in endothelial cells. Inflamm Res. 2009 Aug;58(8):513-21.

[6] Salah-Abbès JB, et al. Tunisian radish extract (Raphanus sativus) enhances the antioxidant status and protects against oxidative stress induced by zearalenone in Balb/c mice. J Appl Toxicol. 2008 Jan;28(1):6-14.

[7] Khaki A, Farnam A, Badie AD, Nikniaz H. Treatment Effects of Onion (Allium cepa) and Ginger (Zingiber officinale) on Sexual Behavior of Rat after Inducing an Antiepileptic Drug (lamotrigine). Balkan Med J. 2012 Sep; 29(3): 236–242.

[8] Akash MS, Rehman K, Chen S. Spice plant Allium cepa: dietary supplement for treatment of type 2 diabetes mellitus. Nutrition. 2014 Oct;30(10):1128-37.

[9] Clifford T, Howatson G, West DJ, Stevenson EJ. The Potential Benefits of Red Beetroot Supplementation in Health and Disease. Nutrients. 2015 Apr; 7(4): 2801–2822.

[10] Zhong J et al. Chemical constituents of Aloe barbadensis Miller and their inhibitory effects on phosphodiesterase-4D. Fitoterapia. 2013 Dec;91:159-165.

[11] Alinejad-Mofrad S, Foadoddini M, Saadatjoo SA, Shayesteh M. Improvement of glucose and lipid profile status with Aloe vera in pre-diabetic subjects: a randomized controlled-trial. J Diabetes Metab Disord. 2015 Apr 9;14:22.

[12] Surjushe A, Vasani R, Saple DG. Aloe Vera: A short review. Indian J Dermatol. 2008; 53(4): 163–166.

[13] Ariana NL, et al. Effect of aloe vera gel on superoxide dismutase (SOD) level in streptozotocin (STZ)-induced diabetic wistar Rattus novergicus liver. 2015. The 3rd ICBS-2013.

[14] Oi Y, et al. Garlic supplementation increases testicular testosterone and decreases plasma corticosterone in rats fed a high protein diet. J Nutr. 2001 Aug;131(8):2150-6.

[15] Ghlissi Z, et al. Antioxidant and androgenic effects of dietary ginger on reproductive function of male diabetic rats. Int J Food Sci Nutr. 2013 Dec;64(8):974-8.

[16] Grzanna R, Lindmark L, Frondoza CG. Ginger--an herbal medicinal product with broad anti-inflammatory actions. J Med Food. 2005 Summer;8(2):125-32.

[17] Frondoza CG, et al. An in vitro screening assay for inhibitors of proinflammatory mediators in herbal extracts using human synoviocyte cultures. In Vitro Cell Dev Biol Anim. 2004 Mar-Apr;40(3-4):95-101.

[18] Ahmed RS, et al. Protective effects of dietary ginger (Zingiber officinales Rosc.) on lindane-induced oxidative stress in rats. Phytother Res. 2008 Jul;22(7):902-6.

[19] Kaul S, Krishnakantha TP. Influence of retinol deficiency and curcumin/turmeric feeding on tissue microsomal membrane lipid peroxidation and fatty acids in rats. Mol Cell Biochem. 1997 Oct;175(1-2):43-8.

[20] Nishiyama T, et al. Curcuminoids and sesquiterpenoids in turmeric (Curcuma longa L.) suppress an increase in blood glucose level in type 2 diabetic KK-Ay mice. J Agric Food Chem. 2005 Feb 23;53(4):959-63.

[21] Aggarwal BB, Gupta SC, Sung B. Curcumin: an orally bioavailable blocker of TNF and other pro-inflammatory biomarkers. Br J Pharmacol. 2013 Aug;169(8):1672-92.

[22] Lantz RC, Chen GJ, Solyom AM, Jolad SD, Timmermann BN. The effect of turmeric extracts on inflammatory mediator production. Phytomedicine. 2005 Jun;12(6-7):445-52.

[23] Song K, Peng S, Sun Z, Li H, Yang R. Curcumin suppresses TGF-β signaling by inhibition of TGIF degradation in scleroderma fibroblasts. Biochem Biophys Res Commun. 2011 Aug 12;411(4):821-5.

[24] Moore MC, Davis SN, Mann SL, Cherrington AD. Acute fructose administration improves oral glucose tolerance in adults with type 2 diabetes. Diabetes Care. 2001 Nov;24(11):1882-7.

[25] Amorim JL, et al. Anti-Inflammatory Properties and Chemical Characterization of the Essential Oils of Four Citrus Species. PLoS One. 2016 Apr 18;11(4):e0153643.

[26] Dreher ML, Davenport AJ. Hass avocado composition and potential health effects. Crit Rev Food Sci Nutr. 2013;53(7):738-50.

[27] Stull AJ, Cash KC, Johnson WD, Champagne CM, Cefalu WT. Bioactives in blueberries improve insulin sensitivity in obese, insulin-resistant men and women. J Nutr. 2010 Oct;140(10):1764-8.

[28] Zhang H, Wang C, Li X, Zhang Y. Effects of *pterostilbene* on treating hyperprolactinemia and related mechanisms. Am J Transl Res. 2016; 8(7): 3049–3055.

[29] Huizhen Cai, et al. Practical Application of Antidiabetic Efficacy of LYCIUM BARBARUM Polysaccharide in Patients with Type 2 Diabetes. Med Chem. 2015 Jun; 11(4): 383–390.

[30] Adams LS, et al. Pomegranate Ellagitannin-Derived Compounds Exhibit Anti-proliferative and Anti-aromatase Activity in Breast Cancer Cells In Vitro. Cancer Prev Res (Phila). 2010 Jan; 3(1): 108–113.

[31] Al-Dujaili, E and Smail, N. Pomegranate juice intake enhances salivary testosterone levels and improves mood and well being in healthy men and women. Endocrine Abstracts. 2012; 28 P313.

[32] Zarfeshany A, Asgary S, Javanmard SH. Potent health effects of pomegranate. Adv Biomed Res. 2014; 3: 100.

[33] Esmaillzadeh A, Tahbaz F, Gaieni I, Alavi-Majd H, Azadbakht L. Cholesterol-lowering effect of concentrated pomegranate juice consumption in type II diabetic patients with hyperlipidemia. Int J Vitam Nutr Res. 2006 May;76(3):147-51.

[34] Lopes de Souza PA, Marcadenti A, Portal VL. Effects of Olive Oil Phenolic Compounds on Inflammation in the Prevention and Treatment of Coronary Artery Disease. Nutrients. 2017 Oct; 9(10): 1087.

[35] Rial SA, Karelis AD, Bergeron K, Mounier C. Gut Microbiota and Metabolic Health: The Potential Beneficial Effects of a Medium Chain Triglyceride Diet in Obese Individuals. Nutrients. 2016 May; 8(5): 281.

[36] Vijayakumar V, et al. Diet enriched with fresh coconut decreases blood glucose levels and body weight in normal adults. J Complement Integr Med. 2018 Feb 20;15(3).

[37] Hyson DA. A comprehensive review of apples and apple components and their relationship to human health. Adv Nutr. 2011 Sep;2(5):408-20.

[38] Kim MS, Kim JY, Choi WH, Lee SS. Effects of seaweed supplementation on blood glucose concentration, lipid profile, and antioxidant enzyme activities in patients with type 2 diabetes mellitus. Nutr Res Pract. 2008 Summer; 2(2): 62–67.

[39] Liu J, et al. Prebiotic effects of diet supplemented with the cultivated red seaweed Chondrus crispus or with fructo-oligo-saccharide on host immunity, colonic microbiota and gut microbial metabolites. BMC Complement Altern Med. 2015 Aug 14;15:279.

[40] Teas J, et al. Dietary seaweed modifies estrogen and phytoestrogen metabolism in healthy postmenopausal women. J Nutr. 2009 May;139(5):939-44.

[41] Hirooka T, et al. Biodegradation of bisphenol A and disappearance of its estrogenic activity by the green alga Chlorella fusca var. vacuolata. Environ Toxicol Chem. 2005 Aug; 24(8):1896-901.

[42] Uchikawa T, et al. Enhanced elimination of tissue methylmercury in Parachlorella beijerinckii-fed mice. J Toxicol Sci. 2011 Jan;36(1):121-6.

[43] Ukhanova M, et al. Effects of almond and pistachio consumption on gut microbiota composition in a randomised cross-over human feeding study. Br J Nutr. 2014 Jun 28;111(12):2146-52.

[44] Liu JF, Liu YH, Chen CM, Chang WH, Chen CY. The effect of almonds on inflammation and oxidative stress in Chinese patients with type 2 diabetes mellitus: a randomized crossover controlled feeding trial. Eur J Nutr. 2013 Apr;52(3):927-35.

[45] Bamberger C, et al. A Walnut-Enriched Diet Affects Gut Microbiome in Healthy Caucasian Subjects: A Randomized, Controlled Trial. Nutrients. 2018 Feb; 10(2): 244.

[46] Garg ML, Blake RJ, Wills RB, Clayton EH. Macadamia nut consumption modulates favourably risk factors for coronary artery disease in hypercholesterolemic subjects. Lipids. 2007 Jun;42(6):583-7.

[47] Şanlier N, Gökcen BB, Sezgin AC. Health benefits of fermented foods. Crit Rev Food Sci Nutr. 2019;59(3):506-527.

[48] Choi IH, et al. Kimchi, a Fermented Vegetable, Improves Serum Lipid Profiles in Healthy Young Adults: Randomized Clinical Trial. J Med Food. 2013 Mar; 16(3): 223–229.

[49] Levkovich T, et al. Probiotic bacteria induce a 'glow of health'. PLoS One. 2013;8(1):e53867.

[50] Wang C, et al. Low-fat high-fiber diet decreased serum and urine androgens in men. J Clin Endocrinol Metab. 2005 Jun;90(6):3550-9.

[51] Chowdhury R, et al. Association of dietary, circulating, and supplement fatty acids with coronary risk: a systematic review and meta-analysis. Ann Intern Med. 2014 Mar 18;160(6):398-406.

[52] Malhotra A, Redberg RF, Meier P. Saturated fat does not clog the arteries: coronary heart disease is a chronic inflammatory condition, the risk of which can be effectively reduced from healthy lifestyle interventions. Br J Sports Med. 2017 Aug;51(15):1111-1112.

[53] Carrillo C, Cavia Mdel M, Alonso-Torre SR. Antitumor effect of oleic acid; mechanisms of action: a review. Nutr Hosp. 2012 Nov-Dec;27(6):1860-5.

[54] Moreno JJ, Carbonell T, Sánchez T, Miret S, Mitjavila MT. Olive oil decreases both oxidative stress and the production of arachidonic acid metabolites by the prostaglandin G/H synthase pathway in rat macrophages. J Nutr. 2001 Aug;131(8):2145-9.

[55] Volek JS, Kraemer WJ, Bush JA, Incledon T, Boetes M. Testosterone and cortisol in relationship to dietary nutrients and resistance exercise. J Appl Physiol (1985). 1997 Jan;82(1):49-54.

[56] Newell-Fugate AE, et al. Effects of coconut oil on glycemia, inflammation, and urogenital microbial parameters in female Ossabaw mini-pigs. PLoS One. 2017 Jul 13;12(7):e0179542.

[57] Chen SR, et al. Icariin derivative inhibits inflammation through suppression of p38 mitogen-activated protein kinase and nuclear factor-kappaB pathways. Biol Pharm Bull. 2010;33(8):1307-13.

[58] Su YS, et al. Icariin promotes mouse hair follicle growth by increasing insulin-like growth factor 1 expression in dermal papillary cells. Clin Exp Dermatol. 2017 Apr;42(3):287-294.

[59] Zhang ZB, Yang QT. The testosterone mimetic properties of icariin. Asian J Androl. 2006 Sep;8(5):601-5.

[60] Gründemann C, et al. Equisetum arvense (common horsetail) modulates the function of inflammatory immunocompetent cells. BMC Complement Altern Med. 2014 Aug 4;14:283.

[61] Chan YS, et al. A review of the pharmacological effects of Arctium lappa (burdock). Inflammopharmacology. 2011 Oct;19(5):245-54.

[62] Navarro-Hoyos M, et al. Proanthocyanidin Characterization and Bioactivity of Extracts from Different Parts of Uncaria tomentosa L. (Cat's Claw). Antioxidants (Basel). 2017 Feb 4;6(1).

[63] Sandoval M, et al. Anti-inflammatory and antioxidant activities of cat's claw (Uncaria tomentosa and Uncaria guianensis) are independent of their alkaloid content. Phytomedicine. 2002 May;9(4):325-37.

[64] Qin B, Panickar KS, Anderson RA. Cinnamon: potential role in the prevention of insulin resistance, metabolic syndrome, and type 2 diabetes. J Diabetes Sci Technol. 2010 May 1;4(3):685-93.

[65] Huang X, Liu Y, Lu Y, Ma C. Anti-inflammatory effects of eugenol on lipopolysaccharide-induced inflammatory reaction in acute lung injury via regulating inflammation and redox status. Int Immunopharmacol. 2015 May;26(1):265-71.

[66] Nagababu E, Rifkind JM, Sesikeran B, Lakshmaiah N. Assessment of Antioxidant Activities of Eugenol by IN VITRO and IN VIVO methods. Methods Mol Biol. 2010; 610: 165–180.

[67] Kandikattu HK. Anti-inflammatory and anti-oxidant effects of Cardamom (Elettaria repens (Sonn.) Baill) and its phytochemical analysis by 4D GCXGC TOF-MS. Biomed Pharmacother. 2017 Jul;91:191-201.

[68] Tadić VM, et al. Anti-inflammatory, gastroprotective, free-radical-scavenging, and antimicrobial activities of hawthorn berries ethanol extract. J Agric Food Chem. 2008 Sep 10;56(17):7700-9.

[69] Shin HS, et al. Hair growth activity of Crataegus pinnatifida on C57BL/6 mouse model. Phytother Res. 2013 Sep;27(9):1352-7.

[70] Hopkins AL, Lamm MG, Funk JL, Ritenbaugh C. Hibiscus sabdariffa L. in the treatment of hypertension and hyperlipidemia: a comprehensive review of animal and human studies. Fitoterapia. 2013;85:84-94.

[71] Adhirajan N, Ravi Kumar T, Shanmugasundaram N, Babu M. In vivo and in vitro evaluation of hair growth potential of Hibiscus rosa-sinensis Linn. J Ethnopharmacol. 2003 Oct;88(2-3):235-9.

[72] Shara M, Stohs SJ. Efficacy and Safety of White Willow Bark (Salix alba) Extracts. Phytother Res. 2015 Aug;29(8):1112-6.

[73] Khayyal MT, El-Ghazaly MA, Abdallah DM, Okpanyi SN, Kelber O, Weiser D. Mechanisms involved in the anti-inflammatory effect of a standardized willow bark extract. Arzneimittelforschung. 2005;55(11):677-87.

[74] Yadav NK, et al. Alcoholic Extract of *Eclipta alba* Shows *In Vitro* Antioxidant and Anticancer Activity without Exhibiting Toxicological Effects. Oxid Med Cell Longev. 2017; 2017: 9094641.

[75] Datta K, et al. Eclipta alba extract with potential for hair growth promoting activity. J Ethnopharmacol. 2009 Jul 30;124(3):450-6.

[76] Thorat RM, Jadhav VM, Kadam VJ. Development and evaluation of polyherbal formulations for hair growth-promoting activity. 2009. Int J Pharm Res. 1:1251-1254.

[77] Begum S, Lee MR, Gu LJ, Hossain J, Sung CK. Exogenous stimulation with Eclipta alba promotes hair matrix keratinocyte proliferation and downregulates TGF-β1 expression in nude mice. Int J Mol Med. 2015 Feb;35(2):496-502.

[78] Ota, Y, et al. Sanguisorba Officinalis Root Extract (SO extract) is a reliable FGF-5 inhibitor. Biochemical and Biophysical Research Communications. 2002;290 (1), 169-176.

[79] Maeda T, Yamamoto T, Youko I. Sanguisorba officinalis Root Extract Has FGF-5 Inhibitory Activity and Reduces Hair Loss by Causing Prolongation of the Anagen Period. Nishi Nihon Hifuka. 2007;69 (1), 81-86.

[80] Serafini M, et al. Plasma antioxidants from chocolate. Nature. 2003 Aug 28;424(6952):1013. Researchers show that consumption of plain, dark chocolate results in an increase in total antioxidant capacity, but that these effects are markedly reduced when the chocolate is consumed with milk or if milk is incorporated as milk chocolate.

[81] Telo S, Halifeoglu I, Ozercanc IH. Effects of Stinging Nettle (*Urtica Dioica L.,*) on Antioxidant Enzyme Activities in Rat Model of Mammary Gland Cancer. Iran J Pharm Res. 2017 Winter; 16(Suppl): 164–170.

[82] Namazi N, Tarighat A, Bahrami A. The effect of hydro alcoholic nettle (Urtica dioica) extract on oxidative stress in patients with type 2 diabetes: a randomized double-blind clinical trial. Pak J Biol Sci. 2012 Jan 15;15(2):98-102.

[83] Roschek B Jr, Fink RC, McMichael M, Alberte RS. Nettle extract (Urtica dioica) affects key receptors and enzymes associated with allergic rhinitis. Phytother Res. 2009 Jul;23(7):920-6.

[84] Schöttner M, Gansser D, Spiteller G. Lignans from the roots of Urtica dioica and their metabolites bind to human sex hormone binding globulin (SHBG). Planta Med. 1997 Dec;63(6):529-32.

[85] Gansser D, Spiteller G. Aromatase inhibitors from Urtica dioica roots. Planta Med. 1995 Apr;61(2):138-40.

[86] Mahdi AA, et al. Withania somnifera Improves Semen Quality in Stress-Related Male Fertility. Evid Based Complement Alternat Med. 2009 Sep 29.

[87] Sharma AK, Basu I, Singh S. Efficacy and Safety of Ashwagandha Root Extract in Subclinical Hypothyroid Patients: A Double-Blind, Randomized Placebo-Controlled Trial. J Altern Complement Med. 2018 Mar;24(3):243-248.

[88] Chandrasekhar K, Kapoor J, Anishetty S. A Prospective, Randomized Double-Blind, Placebo-Controlled Study of Safety and Efficacy of a High-Concentration Full-Spectrum Extract of Ashwagandha Root in Reducing Stress and Anxiety in Adults. Indian J Psychol Med. 2012 Jul-Sep; 34(3): 255–262.

[89] Cha DS, Jeon H. Anti-inflammatory effect of MeOH extracts of the stem of Polygonum multiflorum in LPS-stimulated mouse peritoneal macrophages. Nat Prod Sci. 2009;15:83–89.

[90] Zhang L and Chen J. Biological Effects of Tetrahydroxystilbene Glucoside: An Active Component of a Rhizome Extracted from Polygonum multiflorum. Oxidative medicine and cellular longevity. 2018 Oct.

[91] Park HJ, Zhang N, Park DK. Topical application of Polygonum multiflorum extract induces hair growth of resting hair follicles through upregulating Shh and β-catenin expression in C57BL/6 mice. J Ethnopharmacol. 2011 May 17;135(2):369-75.

[92] Sun YN, et al. Promotion effect of constituents from the root of Polygonum multiflorum on hair growth. Bioorg Med Chem Lett. 2013 Sep 1;23(17):4801-5.

[93] Gao R, et al. Emodin suppresses TGF-β1-induced epithelial-mesenchymal transition in alveolar epithelial cells through Notch signaling pathway. Toxicol Appl Pharmacol. 2017 Mar 1;318:1-7.

[94] Siddiqui MZ. Boswellia Serrata, A Potential Antiinflammatory Agent: An Overview. Indian J Pharm Sci. 2011 May-Jun; 73(3): 255–261.

[95] Oshima M, Gu Y, Tsukada S. Effects of Lepidium meyenii Walp and Jatropha macrantha on blood levels of oestradiol-17 beta, progesterone, testosterone and the rate of embryo implantation in mice. J Vet Med Sci. 2003 Oct;65(10):1145-6.

[96] Shukla KK, Mahdi AA, Ahmad MK, Shankhwar SN, Rajender S, Jaiswar SP. Mucuna pruriens improves male fertility by its action on the hypothalamus-pituitary-gonadal axis. Fertil Steril. 2009 Dec;92(6):1934-40.

[97] Shukla KK, et al. Mucuna pruriens Reduces Stress and Improves the Quality of Semen in Infertile Men. Evid Based Complement Alternat Med. 2010 Mar; 7(1): 137–144.

[98] Ali SF, Hong JS, Wilson WE, Uphouse LL, Bondy SC. Effect of acrylamide on neurotransmitter metabolism and neuropeptide levels in several brain regions and upon circulating hormones. Arch Toxicol. 1983 Jan;52(1):35-43.

[99] Volek JS, Kraemer WJ, Bush JA, Incledon T, Boetes M. Testosterone and cortisol in relationship to dietary nutrients and resistance exercise. J Appl Physiol (1985). 1997 Jan;82(1):49-54.

[100] Azrad M, Turgeon C, Demark-Wahnefried W. Current evidence linking polyunsaturated Fatty acids with cancer risk and progression. Front Oncol. 2013 Sep 4;3:224.

[101] Bajaj JK, Salwan P, Salwan S. Various Possible Toxicants Involved in Thyroid Dysfunction: A Review. J Clin Diagn Res. 2016 Jan; 10(1): FE01–FE03.

[102] Yam D, Eliraz A, Berry EM. Diet and disease--the Israeli paradox: possible dangers of a high omega-6 polyunsaturated fatty acid diet. Isr J Med Sci. 1996 Nov;32(11):1134-43.

[103] Kummerow FA. Interaction between sphingomyelin and oxysterols contributes to atherosclerosis and sudden death. Am J Cardiovasc Dis. 2013; 3(1): 17–26.

[104] Antvorskov JC, Fundova P, Buschard K, Funda DP. Dietary gluten alters the balance of pro-inflammatory and anti-inflammatory cytokines in T cells of BALB/c mice. Immunology. 2013 Jan; 138(1): 23–33.

[105] Lane AR, Duke JW, Hackney AC. Influence of dietary carbohydrate intake on the free testosterone: cortisol ratio responses to short-term intensive exercise training. Eur J Appl Physiol. 2010 Apr;108(6):1125-31.

[106] Frazier TH, DiBaise JK, McClain CJ. Gut microbiota, intestinal permeability, obesity-induced inflammation, and liver injury. JPEN J Parenter Enteral Nutr. 2011 Sep;35(5 Suppl):14S-20S.

[107] Meyers AM, Mourra D, Beeler JA. High fructose corn syrup induces metabolic dysregulation and altered dopamine signaling in the absence of obesity. PLoS One. 2017 Dec 29;12(12):e0190206.

[108] Andreyeva T, Chaloupka FJ, Brownell KD. Estimating the potential of taxes on sugar-sweetened beverages to reduce consumption and generate revenue. Prev Med. 2011 Jun;52(6):413-6.

[109] Chen L, et al. Sugar-sweetened beverage intake and serum testosterone levels in adult males 20-39 years old in the United States. Reprod Biol Endocrinol. 2018 Jun 23;16(1):61.

[110] Aeberli I, et al. Low to moderate sugar-sweetened beverage consumption impairs glucose and lipid metabolism and promotes inflammation in healthy young men: a randomized controlled trial. Am J Clin Nutr. 2011 Aug;94(2):479-85.

[111] Suez J, Korem T, Zilberman-Schapira G, Segal E, Elinav E. Non-caloric artificial sweeteners and the microbiome: findings and challenges. Gut Microbes. 2015;6(2):149-55.

[112] Abou-Donia MB, El-Masry EM, Abdel-Rahman AA, McLendon RE, Schiffman SS. Splenda alters gut microflora and increases intestinal p-glycoprotein and cytochrome p-450 in male rats. J Toxicol Environ Health A. 2008;71(21):1415-29.

[113] Allen NE, Appleby PN, Davey GK, Key TJ. Hormones and diet: low insulin-like growth factor-I but normal bioavailable androgens in vegan men. Br J Cancer. 2000 Jul; 83(1): 95–97.

[114] Simopoulos AP, Salem N Jr. n-3 fatty acids in eggs from range-fed Greek chickens. N Engl J Med. 1989 Nov 16;321(20):1412.

[115] Hites RA, et al. Global assessment of organic contaminants in farmed salmon. Science. 2004 Jan 9;303(5655):226-9.

[116] Aune D, et al. Dairy products, calcium, and prostate cancer risk: a systematic review and meta-analysis of cohort studies. Am J Clin Nutr. 2015 Jan;101(1):87-117.

[117] Maruyama K, Oshima T, Ohyama K. Exposure to exogenous estrogen through intake of commercial milk produced from pregnant cows. Pediatr Int. 2010 Feb;52(1):33-8.

[118] Azzouz A, Jurado-Sánchez B, Souhail B, Ballesteros E. Simultaneous determination of 20 pharmacologically active substances in cow's milk, goat's milk, and human breast milk by gas chromatography-mass spectrometry. J Agric Food Chem. 2011 May 11;59(9):5125-32.

[119] Thompson LU, Boucher BA, Liu Z, Cotterchio M, Kreiger N. Phytoestrogen content of foods consumed in Canada, including isoflavones, lignans, and coumestan. Nutr Cancer. 2006;54(2):184-201.

[120] Nowak DA, Snyder DC, Brown AJ, Demark-Wahnefried W. The Effect of Flaxseed Supplementation on Hormonal Levels Associated with Polycystic Ovarian Syndrome: A Case Study. Curr Top Nutraceutical Res. 2007; 5(4): 177–181.

[121] Demark-Wahnefried W, et al. Flaxseed supplementation (not dietary fat restriction) reduces prostate cancer proliferation rates in men presurgery. Cancer Epidemiol Biomarkers Prev. 2008 Dec;17(12):3577-87.

[122] D'Adamo CR, Sahin A. Soy foods and supplementation: a review of commonly perceived health benefits and risks. Altern Ther Health Med. 2014 Winter;20 Suppl 1:39-51.

[123] Goodin S, et al. Clinical and biological activity of soy protein powder supplementation in healthy male volunteers. Cancer Epidemiol Biomarkers Prev. 2007 Apr;16(4):829-33.

[124] Habito RC, Montalto J, Leslie E, Ball MJ. Effects of replacing meat with soyabean in the diet on sex hormone concentrations in healthy adult males. Br J Nutr. 2000 Oct;84(4):557-63.

Part 5

[1] Gatherwright J, et al. The contribution of endogenous and exogenous factors to male alopecia: a study of identical twins. Plast Reconstr Surg. 2013;131:794–801.

[2] Sonia Haria, "Is your shampoo making your hair thinner?" The Telegraph. Published November 1st, 2017.

[3] Gode V, Bhalla N, Shirhatti V, Mhaskar S, Kamath Y. Quantitative measurement of the penetration of coconut oil into human hair using radiolabeled coconut oil. J Cosmet Sci. 2012 Jan-Feb;63(1):27-31.

[4] Final Report on the Safety Assessment of Sodium Lauryl Sulfate and Ammonium Lauryl Sulfate. Journal of the American College of Toxicology, Volume 2, Number 7. 1983; pp. 127–181.

[5] 12th Report on Carcinogens 2011. US Department of Health and Human Services Public Health Service National Toxicology Program.

[6] Darbre PD, Harvey PW. Paraben esters: review of recent studies of endocrine toxicity, absorption, esterase and human exposure, and discussion of potential human health risks. J Appl Toxicol. 2008 Jul;28(5):561-78.

[7] Gavazzoni DMF. Hair Cosmetics: An Overview. Int J Trichology. 2015 Jan-Mar; 7(1): 2–15.

[8] Gee RH, Charles A, Taylor N, Darbre PD. Oestrogenic and androgenic activity of triclosan in breast cancer cells. J Appl Toxicol. 2008 Jan;28(1):78-91.

[9] Lattanand A, Johnson WC. Male Pattern Alopecia A Histopathologic and Histochemical Study. Journal of Cutaneous Pathology Volume 2. Issue 2, August 1975, Pages 58-70.

[10] Dias M. Hair Cosmetics: An Overview. Int J Trichology. 2015 Jan-Mar; 7(1): 2–15.

[11] Fong P, et al. In silico prediction of prostaglandin D2 synthase inhibitors from herbal constituents for the treatment of hair loss. J Ethnopharmacol. 2015 Dec 4;175:470-80.

[12] Pazyar N, et al. Jojoba in dermatology: a succinct review. G Ital Dermatol Venereol. 2013 Dec;148(6):687-91.

[13] Rele AS, Mohile RB. Effect of mineral oil, sunflower oil, and coconut oil on prevention of hair damage. J Cosmet Sci. 2003 Mar-Apr;54(2):175-92.

[14] Murata K et al. Promotion of hair growth by Rosmarinus officinalis leaf extract. Phytother Res. 2013 Feb;27(2):212-7.

[15] Panahi Y, Taghizadeh M, Marzony ET, Sahebkar A. Rosemary oil vs minoxidil 2% for the treatment of androgenetic alopecia: a randomized comparative trial. Skinmed 2015; 13: 15–21.

[16] William A. Boisvert,et al. Hair growth-promoting effect of Geranium sibiricum extract in human dermal papilla cells and C57BL/6 mice. BMC Complement Altern Med. 2017; 17: 109.

[17] Lee BH, Lee JS, Kim YC. Hair Growth-Promoting Effects of Lavender Oil in C57BL/6 Mice. Toxicol Res. 2016 Apr;32(2):103-8.

[18] Oh JY, Park MA, Kim YC. Peppermint Oil Promotes Hair Growth without Toxic Signs. Toxicol Res. 2014 Dec; 30(4): 297–304.

[19] Koyama T, Kobayashi K, Hama T, Murakami K, Ogawa R. Standardized Scalp Massage Results in Increased Hair Thickness by Inducing Stretching Forces to Dermal Papilla Cells in the Subcutaneous Tissue. Eplasty. 2016; 16: e8.

[20] Kim IH, Kim TY, Ko YW. The effect of a scalp massage on stress hormone, blood pressure, and heart rate of healthy female. J Phys Ther Sci. 2016 Oct;28(10):2703-2707.

[21] English RS Jr, Barazesh JM. Self-Assessments of Standardized Scalp Massages for Androgenic Alopecia: Survey Results. Dermatol Ther (Heidelb). 2019 Mar;9(1):167-178.

[22] Toshitani S, Nakayama J, Yahata T, Yasuda M, Urabe H. A new apparatus for hair regrowth in male-pattern baldness. J Dermatol. 1990 Apr;17(4):240-6.

[23] Tellez-Segura R. Involvement of Mechanical Stress in Androgenetic Alopecia. Int J Trichology. 2015 Jul-Sep;7(3):95-9.

[24] Hsu CK et al. Mechanical forces in skin disorders. J Dermatol Sci. 2018 Jun;90(3):232-240.

Part 6

Sasada T, et al. Chlorinated Water Modulates the Development of Colorectal Tumors with Chromosomal Instability and Gut Microbiota in Apc-Deficient Mice. PLoS One. 2015 Jul 17;10(7):e0132435.

[2] Singh N, Verma KG, Verma P, Sidhu GK, Sachdeva S. A comparative study of fluoride ingestion levels, serum thyroid hormone & TSH level derangements, dental fluorosis status among school children from endemic and non-endemic fluorosis areas. Springerplus. 2014 Jan 3;3:7.

[3] Nickmilder M, Bernard A. Associations between testicular hormones at adolescence and attendance at chlorinated swimming pools during childhood. Int J Androl. 2011 Oct;34(5 Pt 2):e446-58.

[4] Wang ZH, Li XL, Yang ZQ, Xu M. Fluorine-induced apoptosis and lipid peroxidation in human hair follicles in vitro. Biol Trace Elem Res. 2010 Dec;137(3):280-8.

[5] Perumal E, Paul V, Govindarajan V, Panneerselvam L. A brief review on experimental fluorosis. Toxicol Lett. 2013 Nov 25;223(2):236-51.

[6] Yamaguti PM, et al. Effects of Single Exposure of Sodium Fluoride on Lipid Peroxidation and Antioxidant Enzymes in Salivary Glands of Rats. Oxid Med Cell Longev. 2013; 2013: 674593.

[7] Steenland K, Fletcher T, Savitz DA. Epidemiologic Evidence on the Health Effects of Perfluorooctanoic Acid (PFOA). Environ Health Perspect. 2010 Aug; 118(8): 1100–1108.

[8] Johnson PI, Stapleton HM, Mukherjee B, Hauser R, Meeker JD. Associations between brominated flame retardants in house dust and hormone levels in men. Sci Total Environ. 2013 Feb 15;445-446:177-84.

[9] De Long NE, Holloway AC. Early-life chemical exposures and risk of metabolic syndrome. Diabetes Metab Syndr Obes. 2017; 10: 101–109.

[10] Silva E, Rajapakse N, Kortenkamp A. Something from "Nothing" – Eight Weak Estrogenic Chemicals Combined at Concentrations below NOECs Produce Significant Mixture Effects. Environ. Sci. Technol. 2002; 3681751-1756.

[11] Serrano SE, Braun J, Trasande L, Dills R, Sathyanarayana S. Phthalates and diet: a review of the food monitoring and epidemiology data. Environ Health. 2014 Jun 2;13(1):43.

[12] Nicole W. Phthalates in Fast Food: A Potential Dietary Source of Exposure. Environ Health Perspect. 2016 Oct; 124(10): A191.

[13] Chang WH, Li SS, Wu MH, Pan HA, Lee CC. Phthalates might interfere with testicular function by reducing testosterone and insulin-like factor 3 levels. Hum Reprod. 2015 Nov;30(11):2658-70.

[14] Yang CZ, Yaniger SI, Jordan VC, Klein DJ, Bittner GD. Most Plastic Products Release Estrogenic Chemicals: A Potential Health Problem That Can Be Solved. Environ Health Perspect. 2011 Jul 1; 119(7): 989–996.

[15] Tarapore P, et al. Exposure to bisphenol A correlates with early-onset prostate cancer and promotes centrosome amplification and anchorage-independent growth in vitro. PLoS One. 2014 Mar 3;9(3):e90332.

[16] Ribeiro E, Ladeira C, Viegas S. Occupational Exposure to Bisphenol A (BPA): A Reality That Still Needs to Be Unveiled. Toxics. 2017 Sep; 5(3): 22.

[17] Sosnovcová J, Rucki M, Bendová H. Estrogen Receptor Binding Affinity of Food Contact Material Components Estimated by QSAR. Cent Eur J Public Health. 2016 Sep;24(3):241-244.

[18] Camann DE, Zuniga MM, Yau AY, Lester S, Schade M. Concentrations of Toxic Chemicals in PVC Shower Curtains. Epidemiology: 2008 Nov;19(6):S120.

[19] Ruszkiewicz JA, et al. Neurotoxic effect of active ingredients in sunscreen products, a contemporary review. Toxicol Rep. 2017; 4: 245–259.

[20] Darbre PD. Metalloestrogens: an emerging class of inorganic xenoestrogens with potential to add to the oestrogenic burden of the human breast. J Appl Toxicol. 2006 May-Jun;26(3):191-7.

[21] Mutter J. Is dental amalgam safe for humans? The opinion of the scientific committee of the European Commission. J Occup Med Toxicol. 2011 Jan 13;6(1):2.

[22] Gump BB et al. Low-Level Prenatal and Postnatal Blood Lead Exposure and Adrenocortical Responses to Acute Stress in Children. Environ Health Perspect. 2008 Feb; 116(2): 249–255.

[23] Zhai Q, Narbad A, Chen W. Dietary strategies for the treatment of cadmium and lead toxicity. Nutrients. 2015 Jan 14;7(1):552-71.

[24] Abdel Aziz AM, Sh Hamed S, Gaballah MA. Possible Relationship between Chronic Telogen Effluvium and Changes in Lead, Cadmium, Zinc, and Iron Total Blood Levels in Females: A Case-Control Study. Int J Trichology. 2015 Jul-Sep;7(3):100-6.

[25] Jurkowska K, Kratz EM, Sawicka E, Piwowar A. The impact of metalloestrogens on the physiology of male reproductive health as a current problem of the XXI century. J Physiol Pharmacol. 2019 Jun;70(3).

[26] Zwolak I, Zaporowska H. Selenium interactions and toxicity: a review. Selenium interactions and toxicity. Cell Biol Toxicol. 2012 Feb;28(1):31-46.

[27] Takayuki T, Romanas C, Junko T, Mitsuhiro Y, Hiroshi K. Diverse metabolic reactions activated during 58-hr fasting are revealed by non-targeted metabolomic analysis of human blood. Scientific Reports. 2019;9(1).

[28] Wang L, Asimakopoulos AG, Kannan K. Accumulation of 19 environmental phenolic and xenobiotic heterocyclic aromatic compounds in human adipose tissue. Environ Int. 2015 May;78:45-50.

[29] Hodges RE, Minich DM. Modulation of metabolic detoxification pathways using foods and food-derived components: a scientific review with clinical application. Journal of Nutrition and Metabolism, 2015.

[30] Ganesan K, Xu B. A critical review on phytochemical profile and health promoting effects of mung bean (Vigna radiate). Food Science and Human Wellness. 2018 March:11-33.

[31] Szaefer H, Krajka-Kuźniak V, Ignatowicz E, Adamska T, Baer-Dubowska W. Evaluation of the effect of beetroot juice on DMBA-induced damage in liver and mammary gland of female Sprague-Dawley rats. Phytother Res. 2014 Jan;28(1):55-61.

[32] Peterson S, Lampe JW, Bammler TK, Gross-Steinmeyer K, Eaton DL. Apiaceous vegetable constituents inhibit human cytochrome P-450 1A2 (hCYP1A2) activity and hCYP1A2-mediated mutagenicity of aflatoxin B1. Food Chem Toxicol. 2006 Sep;44(9):1474-84.

[33] Laukkanen T, Khan H, Zaccardi F, Laukkanen JA. Association between sauna bathing and fatal cardiovascular and all-cause mortality events. JAMA Intern Med. 2015 Apr;175(4):542-8.

[34] Genuis SJ, Beesoon S, Lobo RA, Birkholz D. Human Elimination of Phthalate Compounds: Blood, Urine, and Sweat (BUS) Study. ScientificWorldJournal. 2012; 2012: 615068.

[35] Rea WJ, Pan Y, Griffiths B. The treatment of patients with mycotoxin-induced disease. Toxicol Ind Health. 2009 Oct-Nov;25(9-10):711-4.

[36] Sears ME, Kerr KJ, Bray RI. Arsenic, cadmium, lead, and mercury in sweat: a systematic review. J Environ Public Health. 2012;2012:184745.

[37] Yang JF, Liu YR, Huang CC, Ueng YF. The time-dependent effects of St John's wort on cytochrome P450, uridine diphosphate-glucuronosyltransferase, glutathione S-transferase, and NAD(P)H-quinone oxidoreductase in mice. J Food Drug Anal. 2018 Jan;26(1):422-431.

[38] Chan YS, et al. A review of the pharmacological effects of Arctium lappa (burdock). Inflammopharmacology. 2011 Oct,19(5):245–254.

[39] Hope, J. A Review of the Mechanism of Injury and Treatment Approaches for Illness Resulting from Exposure to Water-Damaged Buildings, Mold, and Mycotoxins. The Scientific World Journal. 2013, Apr 767482.

[40] Moosavi M. Bentonite Clay as a Natural Remedy: A Brief Review. Iran J Public Health. 2017 Sep; 46(9): 1176–1183.

[41] Botchkarev VA. Stress and the Hair Follicle: Exploring the Connections. Am J Pathol. 2003 Mar; 162(3): 709–712.

[42] Kyung-Hun Son, et al. Relationship between working hours and probability to take alopecia medicine among Korean male workers: a 4-year follow-up study. Ann Occup Environ Med. 2019; 31: e12.

[43] Harb F, Hidalgo MP, Martau B. Lack of exposure to natural light in the workspace is associated with physiological, sleep and depressive symptoms. Chronobiol Int. 2015 Apr;32(3):368-75.

[44] Katuri KK, et al. Association of yoga practice and serum cortisol levels in chronic periodontitis patients with stress-related anxiety and depression. J Int Soc Prev Community Dent. 2016 Jan-Feb;6(1):7-14.

[45] Turakitwanakan W, Mekseepralard C, Busarakumtragul P. Effects of mindfulness meditation on serum cortisol of medical students. J Med Assoc Thai. 2013 Jan;96 Suppl 1:S90-5.

[46] Sinha S, Singh SN, Monga YP, Ray US. Improvement of glutathione and total antioxidant status with yoga. J Altern Complement Med. 2007 Dec;13(10):1085-90.

[47] Field T, Hernandez-Reif M, Diego M, Schanberg S, Kuhn C. Cortisol decreases and serotonin and dopamine increase following massage therapy. Int J Neurosci. 2005 Oct;115(10):1397-413.

[48] Dinan TG, Stilling RM, Stanton C, Cryan JF. Collective unconscious: how gut microbes shape human behavior. J Psychiatr Res. 2015 Apr;63:1-9.

[49] Costa-Pinto FA, Basso AS. Neural and behavioral correlates of food allergy. Chem Immunol Allergy. 2012;98:222-39.

[50] Lange T, Dimitrov S, Fehm HL, Westermann J, Born J. Shift of monocyte function toward cellular immunity during sleep. Arch Intern Med. 2006 Sep 18;166(16):1695-700.

[51] Leproult R, Cauter EV. Effect of 1 Week of Sleep Restriction on Testosterone Levels in Young Healthy Men. JAMA. 2011 Jun 1; 305(21): 2173–2174.

[52] Goh VH, Tong TY. Sleep, sex steroid hormones, sexual activities, and aging in Asian men. J Androl. 2010 Mar-Apr;31(2):131-7.

[53] del Río B, et al. Melatonin, an endogenous-specific inhibitor of estrogen receptor alpha via calmodulin. J Biol Chem. 2004 Sep 10;279(37):38294-302.

[54] Tan DX, Manchester LC, Terron MP, Flores LJ, Reiter RJ. One molecule, many derivatives: a never-ending interaction of melatonin with reactive oxygen and nitrogen species? J Pineal Res. 2007 Jan;42(1):28-42.

[55] Martínez-Campa C et al. Melatonin inhibits both ER alpha activation and breast cancer cell proliferation induced by a metalloestrogen, cadmium. J Pineal Res. 2006 May;40(4):291-6.

[56] Wood B, Rea MS, Plitnick B, Figueiro MG. Light level and duration of exposure determine the impact of self-luminous tablets on melatonin suppression. Appl Ergon. 2013 Mar;44(2):237-40.

[57] Clarke SF, et al. Gut. Exercise and associated dietary extremes impact on gut microbial diversity. 2014 Dec;63(12):1913-20.

[58] Choi J, Jun M, Lee S, Oh SS, Lee WS. The Association between Exercise and Androgenetic Alopecia: A Survey-Based Study. Ann Dermatol. 2017 Aug; 29(4): 513–516.

[59] Hill EE, et al. Exercise and circulating cortisol levels: the intensity threshold effect. J Endocrinol Invest. 2008 Jul;31(7):587-91.

[60] Gomez-Cabrera MC, et al. Oxidative stress in marathon runners: interest of antioxidant supplementation. Br J Nutr. 2006 Aug;96 Suppl 1:S31-3.

[61] Gatherwright J, et al. The contribution of endogenous and exogenous factors to male alopecia: a study of identical twins. Plast Reconstr Surg. 2013;131:794–801.

[62] Richter P, Faroon O, Pappas RS. Cadmium and Cadmium/Zinc Ratios and Tobacco-Related Morbidities. Int J Environ Res Public Health. 2017 Oct; 14(10): 1154.

[63] Trüeb RM. The impact of oxidative stress on hair. Int J Cosmet Sci. 2015 Dec;37 Suppl 2:25-30.

[64] Baig MS, et al. Finasteride-Induced Inhibition of 5α-Reductase Type 2 Could Lead to Kidney Damage—Animal, Experimental Study. Int J Environ Res Public Health. 2019 May; 16(10): 1726.

[65] Wessells H, et al. Incidence and severity of sexual adverse experiences in finasteride and placebo-treated men with benign prostatic hyperplasia. Urology. 2003 Mar;61(3):579-84.

[66] Traish AM, Mulgaonkar A, Giordano N. The Dark Side of 5α-Reductase Inhibitors' Therapy: Sexual Dysfunction, High Gleason Grade Prostate Cancer and Depression. Korean J Urol. 2014 Jun; 55(6): 367–379.

[67] Traish AM, Guay AT, Zitzmann M. 5α-Reductase inhibitors alter steroid metabolism and may contribute to insulin resistance, diabetes, metabolic syndrome and vascular disease: a medical hypothesis. Horm Mol Biol Clin Investig. 2014 Dec;20(3):73-80.